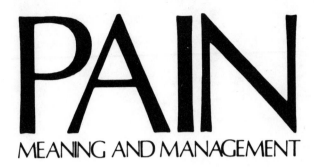

PAIN
MEANING AND MANAGEMENT

PAIN

MEANING AND MANAGEMENT

Edited by

W. Lynn Smith, Ph.D.
Founding Director, Cortical Function Laboratories
Porter Memorial Hospital
and Adjunct Professor of Biological Sciences
University of Denver
Denver, Colorado

Harold Merskey, D.M.
Director of Psychiatric Education and Research
London Psychiatric Hospital
and Professor of Psychiatry
University of Western Ontario
London, Ontario

Steven C. Gross, Ph.D.
Director of Community Learning Centers (Continuing Education)
and Adjunct Assistant Professor of Psychology
Metropolitan State College
Denver, Colorado

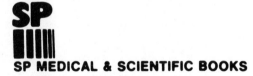

SP MEDICAL & SCIENTIFIC BOOKS

New York • London

SPECTRUM PUBLICATIONS, INC.
175-20 Wexford Terrace, Jamaica, N.Y. 11432

Library of Congress Cataloging in Publication Data

Main entry under title:

Pain, meaning and management.

    Includes index.
    1. Pain. I. Smith, Wallace Lynn, 1922–
II. Merskey, H. III. Gross, Steven C.
RB127.P3324 1980   616'.047   79-21420
ISBN 0-89335-085-0

In memory of Salomon Gross and Reuben Lieberman.

Dedicated to Kevin.

Contributors

DAVID B. BOYD, M.D., F.R.C.P.(C)
Resident in Psychiatry
The University of Western Ontario
London Psychiatric Hospital
Highbury Avenue
London, Ontario

ENRIQUE J.A. CARREGAL, M.D., Ph.D.
Senior Neurophysiologist, Pain Center
City of Hope National Medical Center
Duarte, California

S. GEORGE CARRUTHERS,
M.D., M.R.C.P. (UK), F.R.C.P.(C)
Assistant Professor of Medicine and
   Pharmacology
The University of Western Ontario
   and
Physician
University Hospital
London, Ontario

DAVID H. COY, Ph.D.
Research Service
Veterans Administration Medical Center
New Orleans, Louisiana

BENJAMIN L. CRUE, JR., M.D.
Chairman, Division of Clinical Neurology;
and, Director, Pain Center, City of Hope
   National Medical Center
Duarte, California
   and
Clinical Professor of Surgery (Neurological)
USC School of Medicine
Los Angeles, California

DONALD L. DUERKSEN
Clinical and Research Assistant
Cortical Function Laboratory
Porter Memorial Hospital
Denver, Colorado

G. GAIL GARDNER, Ph.D.
Associate Professor of Clinical Psychology
Assistant Professor of Pediatrics
The University of Colorado Medical School
Denver, Colorado

STEVEN C. GROSS, Ph.D.
Director, Continuing Education; and
Adjunct Assistant Professor
Department of Psychology
Metropolitan State College
Denver, Colorado

CONTRIBUTORS

T.E. HUNT, M.D., F.R.C.P.(C)
Clinical Professor of Medicine
Division of Rehabilitation Medicine
Department of Medicine
University of British Columbia
Vancouver, B.C., Canada
and
Consultant in Rehabilitation Medicine
G.F. Strong Rehabilitation Centre
Vancouver, B.C., Canada

ADA K. JACOX, R.N., Ph.D.
Professor and Associate Dean
School of Nursing
University of Colorado Medical Center
Denver, Colorado

ABBA J. KASTIN, M.D.
Endocrinology Section
Veterans Administration Medical Center
New Orleans, Louisiana
and
Professor, Department of Medicine
Tulane University School of Medicine

BERNARD KENTON, Ph.D.
Senior Neurophysiologist
Pain Center
City of Hope National Medical Center
Duarte, California

H. MERSKEY, D.M.,
F.R.C.P.(C), F.R.C. PSYCH.
Professor of Psychiatry, University
of Western Ontario
and
Director of Education and Research
London Psychiatric Hospital
London, Ontario

J.S. NIELSEN,
M.R.C.S., L.R.C.P., C.R.C.P.(C)
Director of Pain Clinic
Department of Anesthesia
Victoria Hospital
London, Ontario

GAYLE A. OLSON, Ph.D.
Associate Professor
Department of Psychology
University of New Orleans

RICHARD D. OLSON, Ph.D.
Associate Professor
Department of Psychology
University of New Orleans

BERT LINCOLN PEAR, M.D., FACR
Clinical Professor of Radiology
University of Colorado
    Center for Health Sciences
Denver, Colorado
and
Radiologist, St. Joseph Hospital and
    Porter Memorial Hospital
Denver, Colorado

JACK PINSKY, M.D.
Associate Director, Pain Center; and
Psychiatrist in Charge of Pain Unit
City of Hope National Medical Center
Duarte, California

W. LYNN SMITH, PH.D.
Director, Cortical Function Laboratories
Porter Memorial Hospital
Denver, Colorado
White Memorial Medical Center
Los Angeles, California
and
Adjunct Professor of Biological Sciences
University of Denver
Denver, Colorado

Preface

It is ironic that the most common symptom in the field of medicine is also one of the least understood. The present volume offers a survey of many of the most recent relevant issues facing the clinician. The chapters included are original works by noted authorities in their respective fields. Pain, being a topic with many dimensions, is well-represented by authors from a wide range of clinical specialties: neurosurgery, psychiatry, radiology, internal medicine, child psychology, neuropsychology, clinical pharmacology, gerontology, nursing education, endocrinology, and physical medicine. Many of the chapter topics have never before been addressed in a comprehensive way, and certainly not in combination. It is hoped that the reader will be continually reminded of the mind/body interaction involved in pain states. It is the editors' belief that a better understanding of the organic and psychological correlates of pain will result in more successful treatment and management for the patient with pain.

Formal training for most practitioners dealing with the subject of pain is primarily limited to pain's relationship to specific disease processes. The present volume provides a more global understanding of pain and the patient with pain, offering specific treatment approaches based on such understanding.

W. Lynn Smith
H. Merskey
Steven C. Gross

Contents

CHAPTER 1

The Continuing Crisis
In Pain Research

BENJAMIN L. CRUE
BERNARD KENTON
ENRIQUE J.A. CARREGAL
JACK J. PINSKY

INTRODUCTION

Thomas Kuhn (34) has stated that the acquisition of a "paradigm" is a sign of maturity in the development of any scientific field. When the individual scientist can take a paradigm for granted, he need no longer attempt each time to build his field anew, starting from first principles and justifying the use of each concept introduced. Kuhn further points out that normal scientific research is then directed to the articulation of those phenomena and theories inherent in the premises that the paradigm already supplies.

The problems of normal science are described as being "puzzles." What challenges the scientist is the conviction that if he were only skillful enough, he would succeed in solving a puzzle that no one before him had solved. Paradigms are more binding and more complete than any set of rules for research. Yet, according to Kuhn, research under a paradigm must be a particularly effective way for inducing paradigm change. Fundamental novelties of fact and theory, the anomalies of science, are produced inadvertently by the game played under one set of rules, but their assimilation often requires the elaboration of another set.

However, Kuhn observes that the previous awareness of anomaly, the gradual and simultaneous emergence of both observational and conceptual recognition, and the consequent change of a paradigm, often produces resistance. He further states that evidence exists that the same characteristics are built into the nature of the perceptual process itself. In science, novelty emerges only with difficulty, manifest by resistance against the background provided by expectation. However, he minimizes the difficulty of the process by stating that the very fact that a significant scientific novelty so often emerges simultaneously from several laboratories is an index both of the strongly traditional nature of normal science and of the completeness with which that traditional pursuit prepares the way for its own change.

When anomalies in the observations of science proliferate and cannot be reconciled within the rules, or to the basic paradigm, then the significance of the crisis produced is the indication that an occasion for retooling has arrived. Crisis loosens the rules of normal puzzle solving. When the anomaly appears to be more than just another puzzle of normal science, the transition to crisis and to extraordinary science has begun. Even former standard solutions of solved problems can be called into question.

Kuhn also states that the parties to such a revolutionary conflict must finally resort to the techniques of mass persuasion. Furthermore, the price of significant scientific advance is a commitment that runs the risk of being wrong. What occurs during such a scientific revolution is not fully reducible to a reinterpretation of individual and stable data. No ordinary sense of the term "interpretation" can fit the flashes of "intuition" or "imaginative posits" (36) through which a new paradigm is often born. Insofar as the scientist is engaged in normal science, he is a solver of puzzles and not a tester of pardigms. Therefore, paradigm testing occurs only after persistent failure to solve a noteworthy puzzle results in crisis. The transfer of allegiance from one paradigm to another is a conversion experience that cannot be forced. Life-long resistance, particularly from those whose productive careers have committed them to an older tradition of normal science, is not a violation of scientific standard, but an index to the nature of scientific research itself.

Often at issue is just which paradigm should guide future research on presently unsolved problems. Such a decision often rests on faith. The scientific community is a supremely efficient instrument for maximizing the number and precision of problems solved through paradigm change. Inductive reasoning guides the scientist toward the evolution of paradigms that are "useful generalizations of predictive value true to a high degree of probability" (9).

Such a philosophical discussion may be germane to the neurophysiology of today. In a postscript in 1969, Kuhn (34) states that much neural processing takes place between the receipt of a stimulus and the awareness of a sensation. We posit the existence of stimuli to explain our perceptions of the world. Kuhn opposes the attempt to analyze perception as only an interpretative process. Much past experience is embodied in the neural apparatus that transforms stimuli into sensations. We can know stimuli only through elaborate theory.

The present authors consider Kuhn's argument basic to their discussion of the current status of pain research. At the outset, however, we must define our own terms. For our purposes, we might suggest that "sensation" in the human, normally with an intact central nervous system, occurs when we consciously become aware of an external stimulus. "Perception" occurs when we recognize the sensation, and, for all intents and purposes, assign a label to the sensation, and can then again store it in memory. "Conceptualization" occurs when we add the dimension of time and consciously consider the percept in relation to similar past, and imagined future, situations.

Kuhn (35) also stresses the difficulty of communication among scientists committed to different paradigms. While attempting to communicate, such groups often "talk through" each other. The present authors believe that this situation presently prevails in the field of pain research. Despite outstanding attempts by organizations such as the International Association for the Study of Pain, the difficulties in communication concerning pain still exist. At international meetings, the basic scientists are usually present for the first part of the scientific session, then leave; the clinicians often come later, give their reports, and also leave. Attempts at fostering meaningful communication between the various specialties involved in pain research have proved difficult indeed. Dr. Patrick Wall, as the Editor of the new interdisciplinary journal *Pain*, has attempted to improve written communication between the various specialties. But, the "puzzle of pain" (38) continues; and, in the opinion of the present authors, unresolved anomalies between the observations by pain clinicians and the findings of pain researchers represent a continuing serious scientific "crisis." It is time to re-examine some of our paradigms concerning pain. The present authors, however, realize the difficulty of the task that they are asking of both clinicians and neurophysiologists in suggesting a reassessment of their basic underlying paradigms concerning pain. As Thomas Kuhn pointed out, those who break the rules and question the paradigms under which they are carrying out their scientific investigative endeavors, can often be considered to have deserted their particular discipline.

PERIPHERAL NEUROPHYSIOLOGY OF PAIN

Clinical references to pain range far into antiquity (26). The theological aspects of pain were stressed for many centuries. It was only at the end of the 19th century that the study of pain entered a truly scientific phase of inquiry.

Specificity theory, implying the existence of cutaneous nerve endings responding specifically to either mechanical, thermal, or noxious stimuli, has been based largely upon Müller's (42) hypothesis of specific energy (a rather misleading term) and its subsequent development by von Frey (20). Müller proposed a relative stimulus specificity, in which a given nerve fiber would respond preferentially to certain stimuli, although it could be activated by several modalities, in addition to an absolute sensation specificity for each nerve fiber. The concept of end organs specialized to respond to particular types of stimuli was presented by von Frey in 1894. He assumed that the four known cutaneous modalities were subserved by different nerve endings: 1) Ruffini endings for warmth, 2) Krause end-bulbs for cold, 3) free nerve endings around hair follicles and Meissner corpuscles in glabrous skin subserving touch, and 4) free nerve endings for pain.

This assignment of peripheral physiological function to morphologically distinguishable end organs in the skin signaled the ascendancy of the idea of specificity in the entire nervous system. A crucial implication of specificity theory, as presented by von Frey, is the existence of modality-specific central nervous system centers with independent connections from stimulus-specific peripheral end organs.

Acceptance of von Frey's theory, however, was not universal. Goldscheider (22, 23), representing a sizable body of opinion, criticized the inclusion of pain as a single modality, citing the high density of "pain spots" as precluding the possibility of identification of independent warm, cold, or touch spots, which are all pain-sensitive under adequate stimulation. Stating that pain can be elicited by almost any stimulus modality of adequate intensity, Goldscheider proposed a central nervous system origin for pain, based upon intensity and impulse summation.

Other objections to von Frey's theory ranged from its failure to account for the wide range of cutaneous sensory experiences to the inadequacy of his attempts to match specific cutaneous end organs with specific sensations. Anatomical shortcomings in von Frey's concepts were delineated as early as 1905 by Ruffini (47), who emphasized that innumerable types of nerve endings existed intermediate in form between the four entertained by von Frey. Boring (4) also expressed surprise at von Frey's impulsiveness in presenting his anatomical–physiological correlations, since the latter should have been aware that both Goldscheider (22) and Donaldson (18) had previously established the existence of warm and cold spots in the absence of any receptors other than free nerve endings.

Von Frey's failure, however, to correlate function and morphology successfully does not necessarily discredit the idea of specificity. It was Sherrington's (49) view that "The sensorial end-organ is an apparatus by which an afferent nerve fibre is rendered distinctively amenable to some particular physical agent, and at the same time rendered less amenable to, i.e., is shielded from, other excitants. It lowers the value of the limen of stimuli of other kinds." This represented a more meaningful hypothesis upon which to structure a viable theory of cutaneous sensation.

Pattern theory, as espoused by Nafe (43), unlike previous hypotheses based upon clinical observations, was derived from electrophysiological recordings in laboratory animals. Sinclair's (50) description of pattern theory provides a reasonable statement of its content: "For Nafe there need be no specific fibres within a given sense, but only a shifting flux of impulses arriving at the brain dispersed both in time and space. Under such a dispensation each fibre may in its time play many parts, and the fragment of information which it transmits has no sensory significance unless it is integrated with information provided by the remainder of the whole company of fibres in action. Thus activity in a given fibre could at one time contribute towards the experience of pain, cold, or warmth." Pattern theory (51) provides a simple compelling interpretation of the range of cutaneous sensation, but is nonetheless, incapable of denying the existence of stimulus–specific endings.

Throughout the neurophysiological investigations of pain during the 20th century, the concept of pain as a true primary sensation has become an almost universally accepted basic assumption (5, 8, 21, 40, 41). This major premise, underlying neurophysiological pain research, has occasionally been questioned, as was recently done by Perl (45). But, overwhelmingly, pain has been considered neurophysiologically to be a "sensation" (24). This situation is not surprising, since most neurophysiologists' research experience with pain consists of studying acute normal physiologic pain in laboratory animals, whereas clinicians are often confronted with chronic abnormal pain syndromes in their human patients.

Neurophysiologists have been following the rules of the game in attempting to solve the puzzle of pain and have considered pain a sensation when observed from the viewpoint of either specificity or pattern theory. Specificity theory, without question, has been pre-eminent in recent neurophyiological thought. One recent author (25) has concluded that the problem has now been settled in favor of specificity theory. Other investigators have taken a more agnostic approach; but, while not successfully combining specificity, summation, or pattern theory, most researchers have continued to look at pain as a primary sensation. One attempt at such a merger entailed the concept of modulation of input in the region of the dorsal horn, described as a "gating" mechanism. In an outstanding article in *Science* over a decade ago, Melzack and Wall (39) presented their idea of a gate theory of pain in which a relative balance exists between the presumably nonpainful impulses carried in the phylogenetically new, larger, fast fiber system, and the "nociceptive" impulses in the small, phylogenetically older, slow "C" and "A-delta" fiber system.

However, they also considered pain as a sensation with a basically sequential chain of input and began their diagram with impulses approaching the dorsal horn. They did not address the peripheral problem that is so essential to an understanding of this problem. They did not solve the problem of stimulus and sensation relationships at the origin of impulses in the primary afferent peripheral receptor endings where stimuli are first transduced into nerve impulses. It is the present authors' conclusion that some of the neurophysiological concepts underlying Melzack and Wall's modulation of input in the region of the dorsal horn were neurophysiologically incorrect (44), and also that their overall concept is still incomplete (13).

Clinicians who must deal with human chronic pathological pain syndromes have long been unable to accept totally the neurophysiological model of acute pain as a primary sensory modality. For example, in primary trigeminal neuralgia (Tic doulourouex), a light touch stimulus in the proper trigger area of the trigeminal skin distribution may often initiate a lengthy paroxysm of jabbing neuralgic pain (48). Another example is pain existing in the absence of any known peripheral input as in the phantom limb pain syndrome (where there is often phantom limb pain without the other clinical entity of painful stump neuroma).

It has long been the present authors' contention (16) that the neurophysiological mechanism underlying these chronic neuralgic pain states probably represents repetitive firing (i.e., epileptiform activity) in the postsynaptic neurons centrally (37), in the region of the dorsal horn, rather than any imbalance of input from the periphery (10, 15). We believe that with the recording of presumably antidromic activity in the conscious human, synchronous with the tic pain (10), and with the experimental work of researchers such as Black (3), that this concept of an underlying mechanism of epileptiform postsynaptic activity (at least in neuralgic jabbing pain) has been adequately substantiated.

During the last several years, in our neurophysiology pain laboratory at the City of Hope National Medical Center, we have been investigating some of the basic aspects of peripheral stimulation (17) in acute normal physiological animal experiments, since it is believed by the present authors that there is still reason to doubt that pain is a primary sensation. On clinical grounds, we had previously presented (12) our conceptualization of pain as a percept that begins in the central nervous system, probably in the region of the dorsal horn, in response to temporally and spatially patterned input, and which also probably includes a significant degree of peripheral specialization (true specificity). We had presented (see Fig. 1.) a classification of the primary senses based on the concept that the initiating factor in any sensation is the energy in our external milieu that is sufficient to serve as an adequate stimulus. This scheme was compared with the two thousand year old

CLASSIFICATION OF PRIMARY SENSES

CLASSICAL

Presently proposed grouping based on initiating physical source.

1) Vision
2) Hearing
3) Taste
4) Smell
5) Peripheral -(originally "touch")
   a) Cutaneous - touch
      pressure, hot, cold,
      and "pain"
   b) Proprioception

1) Electromagnetic through air
   a) Light
   b) Thermal (by irradiation)
2) Chemical
   a) in air
   b) in liquid
3) Gravity
   a) Proprioception
   b) Vestibular
   c) Mechanical displacement
      from weight bearing surface
4) Mechanical displacement
   through air
5) Cutaneous sensibility
   'a) Mechanical displacement
      by wind, liquid, mass object
   b) Thermal (by conduction)

Fig. 1. Classification of primary senses.

Aristotelian classical pain classification. It will be seen that in the intact skin, *only* two natural forces acting on the tegmentum can be considered as adequate stimuli: mechanical deformation and thermal change.

It must be emphasized that we are not referring to impulses generated by stimuli that are injurious. Tissue damage, both acute (with possible temporary injury potentials) and chronic (where injuries have long since healed, but are presumed to have permanently changed the pattern of response to external forces), are not independently considered in this classification. It is another underlying assumption that pain can be elicited without tissue damage, merely by intensifying an adequate stimulus (i.e., mechanical deformation and thermal change). This has never been proven; but exists as a major neurophysiological premise. This has basic significance, but the language, utilized by both clinicians and neurophysiologists, has caused considerable confusion in this regard. To a clinician a "nociceptor," because of the root derivation of the word, appears to signify a "pain receptor;" yet, when specifically queried, most neurophysiologists familiar with sensory investigation would admit that nociceptor means only a *high threshold* mechanoreceptor or *high threshold* thermoreceptor (52).

We contend that no "pain stimuli" exist in nature, only stimuli that (short of causing tissue damage) cause skin changes adequate to be considered as impulse-initiating stimuli by the process of mechanical deformation or thermal change. They are, thus, not pain stimuli, but only mechanical and thermal stimuli which by analogy are believed (under the parameters of the experiment) probably to be sufficient to elicit a "painful sensation" (or perception?). Thus, in the classical sense, it logically follows that there are no pain endings, pain impulses, or even pain neurons in the mammalian peripheral nervous system.

Since we are at present unable to diagram how the central nervous system initiates, in the region of the dorsal horn, the central percept of pain that can be transmitted upward to conscious conceptualization and an appropriate response, we must be satisfied (13) with the information recorded in Figure 2.

Thus, if the present authors' conceptualization of pain as a central percept is correct, all we can study in the acute laboratory animal experiment, as far as peripheral induction of impulses from external stimuli is concerned, short of tissue damage, is mechanical deformation and thermal change. We initiated our present course of investigating thermal change in mechanoreceptors only when it no longer seemed reasonable to study "pain impulses," and the present authors grew dissatisfied with the concept of pain limited only to a specific sensory modality. Nevertheless, high threshold mechanoreceptors and high threshold thermoreceptors do indeed seem to act as a "nociceptor system" carried in the small fiber C and A-delta system. "Nociceptive input" can be considered, from this standpoint, as a specific anatomic and physiological entity. Subsequent transmission upward, as outlined in the classical sense, has recently been reviewed by Kerr (32). Clinically, the present authors have been concerned with the association between pain and temperature sensation, either hot or cold, in peripheral lesions. Disassociation of pain and temperature does occur in the central nervous system; but, when reported in peripheral neuropathies, such disassociation has usually been incomplete, transient, and usually related with areas of total analgesia or

AFFERENT INPUT
OF
SPINAL DORSAL ROOT

1) Cutaneous

    A. Touch ——▶ Discriminative--fast adapting and fast
conducting. (Hair nets and Meisner
corpuscles) and some slowly adapting
but fast conducting type II mechanoreceptors. Up ipsilateral dorsal
column with some branches to dorsal
horn + to ventral horn for motor
reflex.

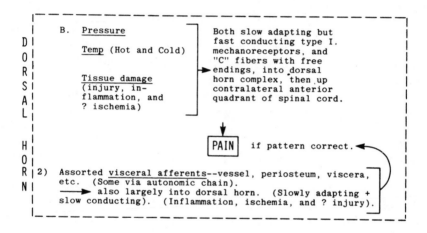

D
O
R
S
A
L

H
O
R
N

    B. Pressure

        Temp (Hot and Cold)

        Tissue damage
        (injury, in-
        flammation, and
        ? ischemia)

Both slow adapting but
fast conducting type I.
mechanoreceptors, and
"C" fibers with free
endings, into dorsal
horn complex, then up
contralateral anterior
quadrant of spinal cord.

PAIN   if pattern correct.

2) Assorted visceral afferents--vessel, periosteum, viscera,
etc. (Some via autonomic chain).
  ——▶ also largely into dorsal horn. (Slowly adapting +
slow conducting). (Inflammation, ischemia, and ? injury).

3) Proprioception portion of gravity sense, largely "non-
adapting" and fast conducting, up ipsilateral dorsal
column to higher CNS (including consciousness) with
branches to dorsal horn + ventral horn for gamma loop
plus for motor reflex + spinocerebellar tracts for
equilibrium (subconscious).

Fig. 2. Afferent input of spinal dorsal root.

anesthesia. We, therefore, speculated that the entire concept of specificity (as
far as any *individual* peripheral fiber is concerned) may be in error. Perhaps
Nafe (43) was correct. If pain is a percept that begins in the central nervous
system, and if only mechanical information and temperature information is
signaled from the periphery, then perhaps many of the individual peripheral
fibers were not unimodal, but polymodal (i.e., bimodal, since there are only
two modalities in the intact skin viewed from the conceptualization). A review

of the literature revealed that many reported putatively unimodal mechano-receptors exhibited sensitivity to temperature change; but, this thermal information had been disregarded and often labeled as "spurious." In 1969, Bessou and Perl (2) developed a thermal classification scheme for *unmyelinated* cutaneous mechanoreceptors. Using mechanical theshold as an independent variable, they reported that "low-threshold mechanoreceptors" displayed increased sensitivity to cooling and a general insensitivity to heat. "Polymodal nociceptors," conversely, were characterized by an opposite response—insensitivity to cooling and an enhanced response to heat. Similar results were reported for *myelinated* fibers by Beck, et al. (1).

All such investigations, however, have been marked by the use of stimulus (or skin) temperature as either an independent or dependent variable. As an independent variable, thermal energy is generally applied to a receptive field, and the spontaneous neural response (or its absence) determines the thermal reactivity of the receptor. When employed as a dependent variable, temperature is correlated with such indepedent variables as nerve fiber conduction velocity or receptor threshold to mechanical stimulation to serve as a basis for receptor classification.

Measured variation of stimulus temperature has rarely been invoked as an experimental technique. Previous workers who have used this technique have limited their investigations to the application of a single temperature value across the range of mechanical stimuli, or of a constant value of mechanical stimulation across a range of thermal stimuli. Since we had predicted (12), based entirely on hypothesis from clinical observation, that perhaps thermal information in the human "rides piggyback" on mechanoreceptive fibers, we decided to add stimulus temperature as a controlled parameter to the mechanical stimulus studies previously performed by Kenton and coworkers (27, 30, 31, 33). This work reveals (28, 29) that using stimulus temperature as a controlled parameter during stimulus response studies of cutaneous mechanoreceptors provides a unique method for determining receptor reactivity to bimodal stimulation. Under these experimental conditions, such reactivity appears to be more prevalent among putatively "unimodal" or "stimulus-specific" end organs than previously accepted.

THERMAL REACTIVITY OF CUTANEOUS MECHANORECEPTORS

Our mechanical stimulator consists of an electromechanical transducer, to which a stylus with a conical-shaped tip (of various tip diameters) is attached. Movements of the shaft extending from the transducer, to which a particular stylus had been connected, were limited to the axial direction and finely regulated by the voltage control potentiometer of an electrical stimulator through a power amplifier. The output range of the transducer lies between

±2.5 mm with a rise time of 7 msec at maximum excursions. Axial displacement of the stylus and the force applied to the tissue undergoing stimulation were monitored by two independent systems of balanced strain gauges attached to the shaft. The strain gauge outputs were recorded by an oscilloscope camera and an XY recorder. Resolution of the strain-gauge output was limited, essentially, only by the resolution of the recording equipment. Receptor responses were filmed simultaneously with the stimulus traces. The entire transducer strain-gauge system was attached to a heavy ball-joint stage mounted on a dual rack-and-pinion system for gross horizontal and vertical positioning. Precise positioning was achieved through micrometer control of the transducer mechanism and the ball-joint stage. (This equipment was developed by Trent Wells, Inc. of South Gate, Calif., in cooperation with the Electronics Instrumentation Division of City of Hope.)

A calibrated heating coil was added to this device and attached to the probe tip to permit the presentation of thermal stimuli to mechanoreceptive fields coinciding with calibrated mechanical stimuli. This bimodal stimulus system permitted the collection of mechanical stimulus-response data with the introduction of stimulus temperature as a controlled parameter.

We then recorded the responses of slowly adapting cutaneous mechanoreceptors to graded, rectangular-shaped mechanical pulses, of 1-sec duration and 10-sec interstimulus interval, ranging in intensity from receptor threshold to maximum response, and applied to the point of maximum sensitivity within the receptive field. Recordings were made from microdissected single dorsal root fibers in the L7 region of the cat.

Analytical techniques employed during these studies included the determination of stimulus-response relationships as well as information transmission functions. The bimodal stimulus series were performed with the probe tip set at preselected elevated temperatures. As previously reported (28, 29), it was found that the stimulus-response data showed that the overwhelming majority of both Type I and Type II mechanoreceptors displayed a change in the average response frequency as a function of stimulus temperature. An unexpected result ensuing from analysis of stimulus-response relationships was the consistency of the normalized response change of the thermally sensitive mechanoreceptors as a function of temperature (under bimodal stimulus conditions). For all such fibers, the mean of the absolute value of this response change per degree centigrade was 0.559 ±0.164. Figure 3 shows the stimulus-response functions of a typical mechanoreceptor at various stimulus temperatures. Examples of bimodal mechanoreceptors as a function of stimulus temperature are shown in Figure 4.

The significance of this study lies in its contribution toward a quantitative determination of the ability of a given "mechanoreceptor" to transmit thermally induced information to the central nervous system. Results of our

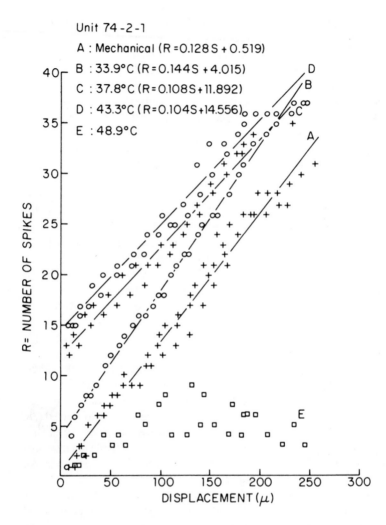

Fig. 3. Response of a moderate-threshold, slowly adapting mechanoreceptor to graded mechanical stimulation of 1-sec duration and 10-sec interstimulus interval, and at various probe-tip temperatures. Linear stimulus–responses relationships comprise the best fitting functions for all data between 25° (room temperature) and 43.3°C (lines A-D). Apparent response breakdown was observed at a probe-tip temperature of 48.9°C (E), above pain threshold. Normal response recurred upon return of the probe tip to room termperature. Line A includes data recorded both before and after the application of thermal stimuli (28, 29).

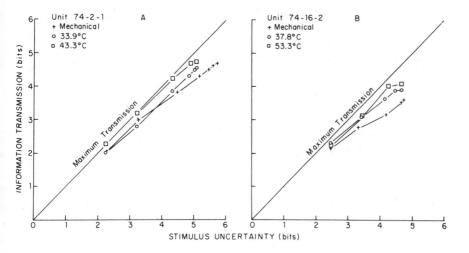

Fig. 4. Effect of thermal stimulation on the transmission of information in two slowly adapting mechanoreceptors. (A) Information transmission functions for the same fiber whose stimulus–response relationships are shown in Figure 3. At the highest value of stimulus uncertainty (i.e., input information) commonly attained during this experiment (5.09 bits), information transmission (i.e., output information) was calculated at 4.73, 4.54, and 4.24 bits, at various probe-tip temperatures. These values correspond to 26-27, 23-24, and 18-19 distinct levels of stimulus discrimination, respectively, and represent increases of 43 and 23% above the number of discrete levels discriminable under purely mechanical stimulation. (B) Similar pattern for another slowly adapting mechanoreceptor. In this case, information transmission values of 4.08, 3.88, and 3.53 bits were achieved at a stimulus uncertainty of 4.68 bits. The corresponding values of 16-17, 14-15, and 11-12 discrete levels represent 46 and 27% increments over the results obtained under mechanical stimulation alone (28, 29).

study bear interesting correlations with the work of Bessou and Perl (2), whose report was limited to unmyelinated fibers, and to that of Beck et al. (1), who studied both unmyelinated and myelinated fiber responses to thermal stimuli. For purposes of comparison, our results are in essential agreement with both of these studies, insofar as experimental techniques overlap. They observed that low-threshold receptors are characterized by heat insensitivity, while moderate-threshold receptors were often marked by heat sensitivity, for both unmyelinated fibers. Their conclusions were based on changes in spontaneous discharge rates as a function of temperature.

Defining "heat-sensitivity" by this criterion alone permitted excellent agreement among their results. However, by employing stimulus temperature as a controlled parameter during *dynamic* studies of receptor response (i.e., via stimulus-response relationships), their classification scheme appears inadequate, since during the present experiments both threshold categories displayed thermal sensitivity under the new criterion with no apparent correlation between receptor threshold and such sensitivity.

The implications of this surprising consistency of response increments among thermally sensitive mechanoreceptors have not yet been explored by the present authors. This phenomenon most probably reflects some underlying uniformity that warrants confirmation and further study.

At this time, the present authors are also unable to substantiate that the temperature information conveyed by mechanoreceptors is utilized centrally by postsynpatic cells. However, to ignore the significance of such thermal information merely because it is transmitted by fibers previously labeled as putatively "mechanoreceptive" seems most unphysiologic.

SUGGESTED PAIN PARADIGMS

The present authors are well aware that a number of valid objections and criticisms might well be aimed at these concepts regarding pain. The concepts of Kuhn may themselves be open to challenge, as has been shown by Popper (46) and Feyerabend (19). We may also be in error to try and define research in pain in terms of a need for new paradigms. However, we obviously believe otherwise.

It must be admitted that much of the difficulty concerning the understanding of pain is a semantic one. Perhaps the main point could have been made by entitling this presentation "Is Pain a Primary Sensation?" We have contended that there are no adequate "pain stimuli" in nature, but only mechanical deformation and thermal change stimuli, that can be applied to the skin. (And specifically, intact skin is implied, with too little work presented on either input changes from acute tissue damage, including skin; or, from abnormalities seen in the input from visceral afferents under pathological conditions.) However, there is both a semantic and a logic problem here. Without much doubt the majority of pain researchers, regardless of background, would admit that pain is not an entity that can be perceived, just as vision and audition are not entities to perceive. Pain is only a word that denotes the act of perception. Thus, a pain receptor cannot exist, and it becomes illogical to point out that one, of course, cannot be specified. Most specifists, of course, must realize that they are concerned with the perception of abnormal tissue change or damage. The question is obviously "Is there a specific system for detecting such injury?" However, even if this concept is realized, there remains the problem of relating this type of "acute injury" (or "specific pain") to the clinical problem of chronic pain, where this acute neurophysiological model may have little role to play beyond a possible original etiological one.

The present authors also realize that they may well be putting too much emphasis on their own findings regarding thermal information carried inward on labeled mechanoreceptors. We have not even ascertained how to substantiate that the central postsynaptic sensory neurones may be able to utilize this input information. We well realize that it serves only as an illustration, as a possible example of a finding that fits well with our previously conceived concept of a generalized or unitary input system. Furthermore, the relationship of this finding to clinical pain certainly remains only a hypothetical one. In constant intractable benign pain, there is no need to postulate any continuing input from an "irritative" peripheral lesion. There is no need for any sustained peripheral "nociceptive" input from a "noxious" stimulus. There really is no one "outside the gate knocking to get in."

There is another interesting possible anomaly, if, indeed, pain research is to be viewed within Kuhn's framework. Research in pain has recently appeared to become a new separate domain of scientific inquiry, rather than a phenomenon of interest to several traditional older domains of research. But, within Kuhn's framework a young science is characterized by multiple simultaneous paradigms; and, rivalries and conflicts of opinion are usually rampant in a young science. Evolutionary and revolutionary processes both emerge as the science matures. The present authors hope that this is happening in the newly combined field of pain research; this may well account for the new and renewed interest in both basic and clinical pain research that has become more evident over the last decade. There is certainly ample evidence that we are still in an infant stage so far as our understanding of pain is concerned, that there is a need for more answers, and that it is clinically important, with chronic pain representing a major unsolved social as well as medical problem. However, the conflicts of opinion over basic pain paradigms, have *not* appeared as rapidly as might have been predicted for a new domain, at least in the view of the present authors. There appear to us to be two main reasons for this finding:

1) Many of those still leading both basic research and clinical treatment in the field of pain, bring to the "new pain domain" their already fixed conclusions (and frank prejudices) which reflect their own original specialized background and training.

Time should take care of this problem.

2) The second reason appears to be the problem of communication within the new domain. This (35) has already been mentioned.

Time will also work to decrease this problem, but, attempts to improve communication should certainly be made, in order, hopefully, to decrease the needed time. This is, in many ways, a reason for the publication of the present article. Hopefully, it may also justify our concluding with two suggested or proposed pain research paradigms, and a discussion of their possible relevance to clinical pain therapy. The present authors are well aware that their proposals contain no new or revolutionary ideas. Indeed, the concepts in both suggested paradigms are over a century old. It is hoped, however, that by reformulating these concepts in this manner we may at least encourage both further discussion and further pain research.

CONCLUSIONS

Proposed Pain Paradigms:

1) Pain (both acute and chronic) is a central perception and *not* a primary sensory modality (sensation). It should be so considered by both clinicians and basic researchers. However, acute pain is usually perceived in response to peripheral input, often related eitiologically to tissue damage.

2) Chronic pain in the human should be considered as a complex phenomenon involving aspects of both present emotional feeling states and past sensory experiences. This includes neuroanatomical, neurochemical, and neurophysiological aspects of both sensation and memory storage, most of which are still largely unexplained. In spite of a peripheral initiating eitiology, with time a central physiological mechanism becomes a self perpetuating generator, perhaps a form of central hypersensitivity based on deafferentiation in many instances, and facilitated in many syndromes by neurone drop out due to aging or CNS pathology. Chronic pain should be considered a CNS phenomenon; and, in most instances there is no need to postulate any continuing peripheral nociceptive input, although any type of input at times can trigger a conscious exacerbation of the pain.

Discussion of Resultants with Clinical Relevance to Pain

1) Consideration of *acute* pain as a percept, and not a primary sensation, may well reorient much present neurophysiological pain research. The peripheral input dilemma between specificity and pattern theory becomes moot as it is put into proper perspective.

2) The understanding of human *chronic* pain, either in the absence of input, or with the stimulus considered only as an initiating trigger of a central mechanism and not as an etiological agent (as in acute pain), shifts the emphasis on understanding and treating the pain from the peripheral stimulus to the "black box" higher in the central nervous system, where it rightly belongs.

3) Clinicians (especially surgeons with scalpels, stereotactic probes, implanted electrical stimulators, and anesthesiologists with needles) might well approach chronic pain in most human syndromes (in the absence of malignant neoplasms) from the standpoint of possible ways to "reprogram the central computer," rather than remaining fixed in the acute pain organic medical model (where they might well have formerly tried to fix some known or presumed peripheral organic abnormality, in a futile attempt to stop some imaginary peripheral "pain" input stimulus that really existed only in the physician's own mind).

4) The psychotherapeutic approach to treatment in chronic benign pain syndromes can thus be interpreted physiologically as an attempt to re-program more favorably the central "black box" computer by subsequent verbal and symbolic inputs as part of a learning process. If the results of the multidisciplinary pain team approach to chronic pain therapy improve with experience and stand up to further investigation, with an acceptable recidivism rate, then perhaps we will see fewer surgical failure patients following multiple operations for chronic benign pain syndromes.

5) Lastly, it is hoped, and to be expected, that the teaching of students about pain will improve significantly. If we admit that there is much yet to be learned about pain, and at present more than one way to view or approach the problem of pain, it should stimulate the iconoclastic spirit in young future pain researchers. Furthermore, it should also instill caution in young future surgeons.

REFERENCES

1. Beck, P.W., Handwerker, H.O., and Zimmermann, M. Nervous outflow from the cat's foot during noxious radiant heat stimulation. *Brain Res.* 67, 373 (1974).
2. Bessou, P. and Perl, E.R. Response of cutaneous sensory units with unmyelinated fibers to noxious stimuli. *J. Neurophysiol.* 32, 1025 (1969).
3. Black, R. Trigeminal pain, in *Pain and Suffering, Selected Aspects.* B.L. Crue, ed. Charles C. Thomas, Springfield, Ill. 1970, ch. 12.
4. Boring, E.G. *Sensation and Perception in the History of Experimental Psychology,* Irvington Pubn., New York, 1942.
5. Casey, K.L. Some current views on the neurophysiology of pain, in *Pain and Suffering, Selected Aspects,* B.L. Crue, ed. Charles C. Thomas, Springfield, Ill. 1970, ch. 15.
6. Casey, K.L. Pain: A current view of neural mechanisms. *Am. Sci.* 61, 194 (1973).
7. Casey, K.L. and Melzack, R. Neural mechanisms of pain: A conceptual model, in *New Concepts in Pain and Its Clinical Management,* E.L. Way, ed. Davis, Philadelphia, 1967.
8. Christensen, B.N. and Perl, E.R. Spinal neurons specifically excited by noxious or thermal stimuli: Marginal zone of the dorsal horn. *J. Neurophysiol.* 33, 293 (1970).
9. Crue, B.L. Some philosophical considerations of pain-suggestion, euthanasia, and free will, in *Pain, Research and Treatment,* B.L. Crue, ed. Academic Press, New York, 1975, ch. 35.
10. Crue, B.L., Carregal, E.J.A., and Todd, E.M. Neuralgia—Discussion of central mechanisms. *Bull. L.A. Neurol. Soc.* 29, 107 (1964).

11. Crue, B.L. and Carregal, E.J.A. Post-synaptic repetitive neurone discharge in neuralgic pain. Presented at International Symposium on Pain, May 21-26, 1973, Seattle, Washington. Published in, *Advances in Neurology*, vol.4. J. Bonica, ed. Raven Press, New York, pp. 643-650.

12. Crue, B.L. and Carregal, E.J.A. Pain begins in the dorsal horn—With a suggested classification of the primary senses, in *Pain—Further Observations from the City of Hope*. B.L. Crue, ed. Academic Press, New York, 1975, ch. 3.

13. Crue, B.L., Kenton, B., and Carregal, E.J.A. Neurophysiology of Pain—Speculation concerning the possibility of a unitary peripheral cutaneous input system for pressure, hot, cold, and tissue damage: Discussion of relationship to pain (specificity theory as an evolving mechanism superimposed on pattern theory). Presented at First World Congress on Pain, Florence, Italy, September 7, 1975. Published in, *Bull. L.A. Neurol. Soc.* 41, 13 (1976).

14. Crue, B.L., Todd, E.M., and Carregal, E.J.A. Cranial neuralgia—Neurophysiological considerations, in *Handbook of Clinical Neurology*, vol. 5. P.J. Vinken and G.W. Bruyn, eds. North-Holland Pub. Co., Amsterdam, 1968, ch. 27.

15. Crue, B.L., Todd, E.M., and Carregal, E.J.A. Observations on the present status of the compression procedure in trigeminal neuralgia, in *Pain and Suffering, Selected Aspects*. B.L. Crue, ed. Charles C. Thomas, Springfield, Ill. 1970, ch. 7.

16. Crue, B.L., Shelden, C.H., Pudenz, R.H., and Freshwater, D.B. Observations on the pain and trigger mechanisms in trigeminal neuralgia. *Neurology* 6, 196 (1956).

17. Dethier, V.G. A surfeit of stimuli: A paucity of receptors. *Am. Sci.* 59, 706 (1971).

18. Donaldson, H.H. On the temperature sense. *Mind* 10, 399 (1885).

19. Feyerabend, P.K. Consolations for the specialist, in *Criticism and the Growth of Knowledge*, I. Lakatos and A.E. Musgrave, eds. Cambridge Univ. Press, England, 1970.

20. von Frey, M. Beiträge zur Physiologie des Schmerzsinns. *Ber Sachs. Ges-amte, Wiss. Math-Phys. Clone* 46, 185 (1894).

21. Georgopoulous, A.P. Functional properties of primary afferent units probably related to pain mechanisms in primate glabrous skin. *J. Neurophysiol.* 39, 71 (1976).

22. Goldscheider, A. *Die Lehre von den spezifischen Energien der Sinnerszerven*. Berlin, 1881.

23. Goldscheider, A. *Das Schmerzproblem*. Berlin, 1916.

24. Granit, R. *Receptors and Sensory Perception*. Yale Univ. Press, New Haven, Conn., 1955.

25. Iggo, A. Introduction, in *Handbook of Sensory Physiology*, Vol. II. *Somato-sensory systems*. W.R. Lowenstein, ed., Springer Verlag, Berlin, 1973.

26. Keele, K.D. *Anatomies of Pain*. Blackwell Press, Oxford, England, 1957.

27. Kenton, B. A critique on neurophysiological psychophysical correlations, in *Further Observations on Pain from the City of Hope*. B.L. Crue, ed. Academic Press, New York, 1975, ch. 8.

28. Kenton, B., Crue, B.L., and Carregal, E.J.A. Quantitative measures of the thermal reactivity of cutaneous mechanoreceptors. *Neurosci. Lett.* 1, 321 (1975).

29. Kenton, B., Crue, B.L., and Carregal, E.J.A. The role of cutaneous mechanoreceptors in thermal sensation and pain. *Pain* 2, 119 (1976).

30. Kenton, B. and Kruger, L. Information transmission in slowly adapting mechanoreceptors. *Exp. Neurol.* 31, 114 (1971).

31. Kenton, B., Kruger, L., and Woo, M. Two classes of slowly adapting mechanoreceptor fibers in reptile cutaneous nerve. *J. Physiol.* 212, 21 (1971).

32. Kerr, F.W.L. Neuroanatomical substrates of nociception in the spinal cord. *Pain* 1, 325 (1975).

33. Kruger, L. and Kenton, B. Quantitative neural and psychophysical data for cutaneous mechanoreceptor function. *Brain Res.* 49, 1 (1973).

34. Kuhn, T.S. *The Structure of Scientific Revolutions*. Univ. of Chicago Press, Chicago, Ill.,

1962. (2nd ed., 1970).
35. Kuhn, T.S. Reflections on my critics, in *Criticism and the Growth of Knowledge*. I. Lakatos and A.C. Musgrave, eds. Cambridge Univ. Press, England, 1970.
36. Lakatos, I. and Musgrave, A.E. *Criticism and the Growth of Knowledge*. Cambridge Univ. Press, England, 1970.
37. Livingston, W.K. *Pain Mechanisms, a Physiologic Interpretation of Causalgia and its Related States*. Macmillan, New York, 1944.
38. Melzack, R. *The Puzzle of Pain*. Basic Books, New York, 1973.
39. Melzack, R. and Wall, P.D. Pain Mechanisms: A new theory. *Science* 150, 971 (1965).
40. Melzack, R. and Wall, P.D. Gate control theory of pain, in *Pain*. A. Soulairac, J. Cahn, and J. Charpentier, eds. Academic, New York, 1968.
41. Melzack, R. and Wall, P.D. Psychophysiology of pain. *Int. Anesthesiol. Clin.* 8, 3 (1970).
42. Müller, J. *Handbuch der Physiologie des Menschen*. Coblenz, 1838.
43. Nafe, J.P. The psychology of felt experience. *Am. J. Psychol.* 39, 367 (1927).
44. Nathan, P.W. The gate-control theory of pain—A critical review. *Brain* 99, 123 (1976).
45. Perl, E.R. Is pain a specific sensation? *J. Psychiatr. Res.* 8, 273 (1971).
46. Popper, K.R. *Conjectures and Refutations: The Growth of Scientific Knowledge*. Harper & Row, New York, 1963.
47. Ruffini, A. Les dispositifs anatomiques de la sensibilite cutanee sur les expansions nerveuses de la peau chez l'homme et quelques autres mammiferes. *Rev. Gen. Histo.* 1, 421 (1904-5).
48. Shelden, C.H., Pudenz, R.H., Freshwater, D.B., and Crue, B.L. Compression rather than decompression for trigeminal neuralgia. *J. Neurosurg.* 12, 123 (1955).
49. Sherrington, C.S. Cutaneous sensations, in *Textbook of Physiology*, vol. 2. E.A. Schäfer, ed., Edinburgh, 1900, pp. 920-1001.
50. Sinclair, D.C. Cutaneous sensation and the doctrine of specific energy. *Brain* 78, 584 (1955).
51. Sinclair, D. *Cutaneous Sensation*. Oxford Univ. Press, England, 1967.
52. Zimmermann, M. Neurophysiological models for nociceptors, pain, and pain therapy, in *Advances in Neurosurgery*, vol. 3. Pengholy, Brock, Homer, Klinger, and Spoerri, eds., Springer-Verlag, Berlin, 1975.

CHAPTER 2

The Opioid Neuropeptides Enkephalin and Endorphin and their Hypothesized Relation to Pain

GAYLE A. OLSON
RICHARD D. OLSON
ABBA J. KASTIN
DAVID H. COY

INTRODUCTION

Research during the last decade has provided us with much new and startling information concerning the interrelationship of pituitary and hypothalamic hormones and neuropeptides on the one hand and behavior and brain functions on the other. Of particular interest here is a subset of that research dealing with the endogenous opioid or morphine-like peptides that have recently been discovered and characterized in the brain: the brain's own morphine.

OPIATE RECEPTORS

It has been known for a long time that morphine and other opiates produce profound behavioral and pharmacological effects, such as euphoria, analgesia, dependence, and respiratory depression. Only recently was it discovered that there are, in the brain and certain other parts of the body, highly stereospecific receptors for the alkaloids from the opium poppy. Goldstein et al. (42) reported the discovery of such receptors in the mouse brain, thereby presenting not only a finding that would initiate the search for an understanding of the fundamental mechanisms of action of the opiate narcotics, but also provide a methodology for doing so. Refinements of this procedure by Simon et al. (115), Pert and Snyder (99), and Terenius (121) provided improved assay methods to further research in the area. Stereospecific binding and naloxone reversibility (reversal of the effects by an opiate antagonist, such as naloxone) have become criteria for determining these receptors.

Numerous investigators have attempted to discover the distribution of these opiate receptors. Opiate receptors have been found in a wide range of vertebrates, including fish, amphibians, reptiles, birds, and mammals (95), but no such receptors were discovered in any invertebrates. They also found that opiate receptor binding has similar characteristics in all vertebrate species studied, suggesting the possibility of a common physiological function for these receptors independent of the response to opiates. A neurotransmitter role was postulated, although the inability to find opiate receptors in invertebrates, in spite of the fact that they have the same neurotransmitters as vertebrates, cast some doubts on this hypothesis. Pert et al. did suggest the possibility of a different type of synaptic function, unique to vertebrates, associated with the opiate receptors.

Localization of these receptors within a species has also been studied. The distributions of the receptors corresponded in part to certain pathways in the brain that are known to be pain pathways, thus suggesting that these receptors and opiate-like substances (either exogenous or endogenous) were related to pain and its transmission in the nervous system. In monkeys and human beings the number of opiate receptors varied dramatically (70). The amygdala contained the greatest amount of receptor binding, with the anterior portion having the most receptors. The hypothalamus and thalamus had the next most. No receptors were found in the cerebellum or in parts of the cortex. The lack of opiate receptors in the cerebellum has been confirmed (95) in studies with chickens, fish, rats, monkeys, and human beings. The medial periventricular-periaqueductal gray of the midbrain and diencephalon as well as a more lateral distribution of the midbrain, including the lateral reticular nucleus, substantia nigra, red nucleus, and thalamus, also have been shown to contain a large number of receptors (94); these two areas coincide with areas thought to mediate pain.

In the rat, similar distributions have been shown (118). The amygdala has the most receptors, but only slightly more than the periaqueductal gray of the midbrain, hypothalamus, and medial thalamus. Receptor binding was also found to be high in the caudate nucleus. Within the cerebral cortex there are areas with no or very low numbers of receptors, such as the white matter, and areas with considerable amounts of receptor binding; the frontal cortex binds more than four times the amount of opiates as that of the precentral and postcentral gyri and occipital pole, thus demonstrating the variability within the cortex. The spinal cord and cerebellum, like the white matter of the cortex, have few, if any, receptors.

The substantia gelatinosa of the spinal cord of cats has been shown to have a particularly high number of opiate receptors (26), as have the olfactory regions in fish, chickens, sharks, monkeys, and human beings (95). There are other areas which have been shown to contain such receptors, too, including the guinea pig ileum (99) and the mouse vas deferens (50), both of which are systematically used to study opiate receptor binding. Pert and Synder (99) found that the opiate receptor is confined to nervous tissue, thus further suggesting that these receptors are related in some way to neural transmission and perhaps the transmission of pain.

The same receptors tend to bind both strong opiate agonists and pure opiate antagonists, with the two competing for the binding sites, while partial or mixed agonist-antagonists appear to work on these same receptors for antagonist action, but on other receptors for agonist action (22). Pure opiate antagonists (such as naloxone) differ chemically from agonists only in the substitution of an N-allyl, N-cyclopropyl, or a related group for the N-methyl of agonists (118). The mixed agonist-antagonists are of some interest because they are thought to be relatively nonaddicting analgesics. Pentazocine is an example of such analgesics that is already clinically marketed (118).

Since opiate agonists and antagonists are so similar and since they compete for the same receptors, there must be some mechanism postulated to account for the differential binding of these agents at any specific time. The presence or absence of sodium, or at least the sodium concentration, affect the binding such that sodium enhances antagonist, but decreases agonist, binding (97). The ability to enhance antagonist binding is not a general characteristic of all cations or high ionic strength, but is a property of sodium ions (116). The increase in antagonist binding results from enhancement of affinity, not unmasking of new binding sites, with the changes in binding affinity being accounted for by changes in dissociation or association rate (116).

Recently Jacquet et al. (59) provided evidence for two distinct classes of receptors that mediate morphine effects. There are receptors with a high degree of stereospecificity, which are blocked by naloxone and which mediate analgesia; their endogenous ligands (naturally occurring substances which bind specific receptors), are endorphins. The other kind has a low degree of stereospecificity and is not blocked by naloxone. This latter variety mediates hyperexcitability and explosive motor behavior, similar to withdrawal symptoms. It was speculated that these latter receptors may play a significant role in opiate dependence, while the former play a role in pain perception.

Creese and Snyder (24) compared the affinities of opiate agonists, antagonists, and agonist-antagonists for binding sites in the guinea pig ileum and the pharmacological potency of the agents. Receptor binding correlated very well with pharmacological potency. A similar study (86) comparing the apparent affinity of various opiate agonists and antagonists for the binding sites in the rat brain and their known pharmacological activity also found a close correlation between the two variables. Thus, measures of opiate binding are considered to be good indices of the pharmacological activity of the agents and can be used as independent measures of their potency.

ISOLATION OF ENDOGENOUS OPIOID SUBSTANCES

It seemed very unlikely that such highly stereospecific receptors should have developed in vertebrate animals solely to interact with plant-produced substances. Instead, it is more reasonable to assume that the receptors have some physiological function in the organism independent of plant opiates and that the opiate receptors were really receptors for endogenous morphine-like ligands. With this premise, Hughes (55) attempted to find such an endogenous factor. Extracts were taken from the brains of rabbits, guinea pigs, rats, and pigs and were purified. A substance of low molecular weight was identified, which had an inhibitory effect on neurally evoked contractions of the tissue of the mouse vas deferens and guinea pig myenteric plexus, which were known to possess morphine receptor sites. The inhibitory action was reversed by the opiate antagonist, thereby confirming its action on opiate receptors per se. Observations of the pharmacological activity of the substance and its characteristics led Hughes to suggest that it was a peptide.

Hughes (55) found that this substance, at that time still unnamed but now called enkephalin, was unevenly distributed in the brain, with the highest concentrations occurring in the striatum, midbrain, pons, and medulla. No activity was found in extracts of the cerebellum, lungs, and liver. There appeared to be a general correspondence between the occurrence of this substance in the brain and the opiate receptor binding sites already mapped, although a detailed study of this aspect was not carried out. It was suggested that this newly isolated endogenous compound might form part of a central pain suppressive system, considering all of its morphine-like properties.

Terenius and Wahlstrom (123) also attempted to discover an endogenous ligand for the opiate receptor sites. They processed extracts from rat brain and found an active factor with receptor blocking activity. Extracts from all areas of the brain, except the cerebellum, contained this substance, which was found to interact with dihydromorphine in a competitive and reversible fashion. This fraction was thought to be a peptide, since, among other characteristics, it was heat stable, polyionic, and had an apparent molecular weight of 1000–1200 daltons. The authors suggested that the endogenous factor might have physiological significance during the development of opiate tolerance or under the conditions of chronic pain. It might well be that chronic pain produces changes in the concentrations of these substances in the brain.

Terenius and Wahlstrom (122) identified a fraction of human cerebrospinal fluid which was found to show affinity for opiate receptors. This factor behaved in a similar fashion to morphinomimetic analgesics and not like narcotic antagonists, so they called it morphine-like factor (MLF). The level of MLF varied between individuals and was lower in patients with trigeminal neuralgia, suggesting further its relation to pain and its perception. The MLF was also found to be similar to the substance they had isolated from brain extracts, although the cerebrospinal fraction seemed to be considerably less complex than the corresponding fraction from brain extracts. Their MLF had characteristics suggesting that it might be a peptide.

ENKEPHALINS

Hughes et al. (57) described the purification and properties of a peptide of low molecular weight (800-1200 daltons) that was extracted from the pig brain. This substance, which they named enkephalin, acted as an agonist at opiate receptor sites and its action was prevented by a wide range of narcotic antagonists. The exact amino acid seqeunce was not discovered at that time, but some of its composition was determined. It was not known whether or not there was only a single peptide with such properties. They did discover that enkephalin is rapidly destroyed by tissue extracts, making its study difficult; an effective means of preventing such inactivation was needed to facilitate research involving it. The authors speculated that it seemed unlikely that enkephalin was solely concerned with the modulation of pain perception. Its wide distribution in the brain and presence in the guinea pig ileum suggested a broader neurochemical role, whose nature was unknown.

Hughes and his associates (56) identified the amino acid sequence of two related pentapeptides from the pig brain with potent opiate agonist activity as enkephalins. There were two varieties, based on the amino acid sequence: methionine-enkephalin (H-Tyr-Gly-Gly-Phe-Met-OH) and leucine-enkephalin (H-Tyr-Gly-Gly-Phe-Leu-OH). Leu-enkephalin has only half the potency of met-enkephalin in the vas deferens and only one-fifth of that of met-enkephalin in the guinea pig ileum. In addition, met-enkephalin is twenty times more potent that normorphine in the vas deferens and is equipotent with normorphine in the guinea pig ileum. It was estimated that the ratio of methionine-enkephalin (met-enkephalin) to leucine-enkephalin (leu-enkephalin) in the pig brain was 3 or 4 to 1. This last finding was in contrast to that of Simantov and Snyder (114), who found that the bovine brain contains four times as much leu-enkephalin as met-enkephalin. Thus, there appear to be species differences in the brain content of these enkephalins.

Further investigations of these newly found endogenous morphine-like factors produced more information about them. Pasternak et al. (91) found that, in rat and calf brains, enkephalin has a regional distribution correlating with that of opiate receptors, as Hughes (55) had earlier suggested. The highest levels of this factor were found in the caudate and a negligible amount was found in the cerebellum, as expected. In binding assays, the factor acted as an opiate agonist, like morphine. The investigators described the localization and characteristics of the substance. In a similar study, Teschemacher et al. (125) described a method for extraction from bovine pituitary of a substance that shows several opiate characteristics, including inhibiting the electrically induced firing of the guinea pig ileum and the mouse vas deferens. It inhibited the binding of opiate agonists and antagonists and was reversed by naloxone.

A high content of enkephalin in the striatum was reported by Smith et al. (117) and a dense network of enkephalin-containing neurons was found in the striatum by Elde et al. (29). These observations suggested to Pollard et al. (101) the possible connection between the enkephalinergic neurons and the dopaminergic fibers ending in the striatum. They studied the effect of chemical or mechanical interruption of the nigrostriatal bundle. They found that both the regional distribution of leu-enkephalin binding sites and their number were affected by this damage, with the decrease in the number sites, supporting the assumption that enkephalinergic neurons terminate presynaptically on dopaminergic nerve terminals in the striatum. The authors speculated that a major physiological function of enkephalins could be to mediate presynaptic inhibitions of a variety of neuronal systems in the central nervous system.

More detailed descriptions of the biochemical and physiochemical properties of the enkephalins followed these original descriptions of their activities. Garbay-Jaureguiberry et al. (33) proposed a preferential conformation of met-enkephalin in DMSO-D_6 solution. This conformation was characterized by a highly folded secondary structure with a β-I turn involving an H bond between the CO of the Tyr residue and the NH of the Phe residue. This conformation was somewhat different from that advanced by Bradbury et al. (11), who also suggested the importance of the β turn. Horn and Rodgers (53) also proposed a model with a β turn, since that model was consistent with certain of the exogenous opiate structure-function relationships. Jones et al. (64) suggested that the apparent discrepancies reported in the literature might be due to the existence of two forms, cationic and zwitterionic, of met-enkephalin. The proton magnetic resonance (PMR) parameters of these two forms indicate different conformations, with a 2-5 β-I turn in the zwitterionic, but not the cationic, form.

The results of an extensive study by Agarwal et al. (1) provided little support for a model of leu-enkephalin having a similar structure to that of met-enkephalin in terms of having either an α-helical or β turn. Thus, the β turn may not be characteristic of the enkephalins (64) and may not be a necessary structure for receptor conformation.

Hughes (55), in his early work, demonstrated that the enkephalins were subject to rapid deactivation when exposed to tissue homogenates and purified enzyme preparations such as carboxypeptidase-A and leucine aminopeptidase. Hambrook et al. (49) found that the deactivation of enkephalins in rat and human plasma takes place through the cleavage of the Tyr-Gly bond. The localization, nature, and specificity of the possible enzyme system responsible for the cleavage have not been determined.

In addition to identifying the natural enkephalins, Hughes et al. (56) also synthesized both forms of enkephalin. Although a detailed pharmacology of the synthetic peptides was not presented at that time, the investigators did indicate a very close agreement between the pharmacological activities of the natural and synthetic peptides when tested on the guinea pig ileum and the mouse vas deferens. On the basis of this close correspondence, the investigators concluded that their assigned structures for the two enkephalins were correct. They further suggested that the discovery of these endogenous pentapeptides allows the testing of the hypothesis that these peptides act as neurotransmitters or that they play a physiological role in the perception of pain.

Since the effects of enkephalin were short-lived and weak, due in part to a rapid degradation, a search began for analogs with greater stability. Coy et al. (23) reported the synthesis by solid-phase methods and testing of a series of D-amino acid-substituted analogs of met-enkephalin. The analogs were tested for their abilities to inhibit electrically evoked contractions of mouse vasa deferentia and to compete with tritiated enkephalin for opiate receptors on particulate fractions isolated from homogenates of rat brain. [D-Ala²]-enkephalin and [D-Ala²]-enkephalin amide were found to be the most potent peptides in both assay systems. In comparison, [D-Met⁵]-, [D-Tyr¹]-, [D-Leu²]-, [D-Phe²]-, [D-Ala³]-, and [D-Phe⁴]-enkephalin had very low rates of activity. The stabilization of the β-bend conformation of met-enkephalin by the substitution of the D-alanine in position 2 of the peptide chain was thought by the authors to contribute to the high activities of the [D-Ala²]-analogs.

At about the same time, Pert et al. (98) also reported the synthesis of [D-Ala²]-met-enkephalinamide. They reported that the analog bound to opiate receptors almost as tightly as the natural substance. Since it was found not to be susceptible to degradation by brain enzymes, the analog in low doses caused profound, long-lasting, morphine-like analgesia when microinjected into the rat brain. No analgesia resulted from intravenous injection, leading the authors to conclude, perhaps prematurely, that the analog does not cross the blood-brain barrier.

A different series of five enkephalin analogs was synthesized using fragment condensation methods and tested for analgesic activity by Roemer et al. (108). Two of the analogs exhibited significant analgesic activity after oral and parenteral administration, as well as intracerebroventricular, intravenous, and subcutaneous administration. Mice, rats, rhesus monkeys, and rabbits were studied in the various tests conducted. One of the analogs, designated 33-824, was found to be extremely potent and long-lasting, even after systemic administration. It produced a marked catatonia characterized by muscular rigidity and immobility lasting at least 2 hr.

ENDORPHINS

As more information became available about the characteristics of the enkephalins, it became apparent that there were several other, larger, naturally occurring peptides that also shared similar pharmacological properties. The relationship of the enkephalins to β-lipotropin suggested that further research with that hormone might be productive in discovering these hypothesized larger peptides. Bradbury et al. (11) noted that the amino acid sequence of enkephalin is identical to that at the NH_2-terminus of β-lipotropin C fragment, a peptide they had previously discovered in substantial quantity in porcine pituitary (10). The C-fragment represented the 61-91 sequence. Later in Bradbury's laboratory (12), the C-fragment was shown to produce strong and lasting analgesia upon intraventricular infusion in the rat. Its analgesic properties were compared with those of three synthetic derivatives of met-enkephalin, with the C-fragment being approximately 50 times more potent than the enkephalin analogs. The investigators concluded that it is the length of the C-fragment rather than the resistance of its N-terminal pentapeptide to degradation that determines the analgesic properties.

Graf et al. (44) also studied the morphine-like effects of enkephalins and other lipotropin fragments, including the 61-91 sequence which Bradbury had called the C-fragment, but which is now commonly referred to as β-endorphin. The highest opiate activity for the fragments was exhibited by β-endorphin for both in vivo and in vitro measures, with little in vivo activity being found for met-enkephalin.

Attacking the problem from another angle, Chretien et al. (20) isolated peptides with opiate activity from sheep and human pituitaries which were of identical size, composition, and N-terminal residue to the carboxyl-terminal portion 61-91 of β-lipotropin, namely β-endorphin. These peptides exhibited morphine-like activity in the mouse vas deferens. β-lipotropins from both species exhibited much lower potency than the newly isolated fragments in the same bioassay. The investigators suggested that the findings favored the hypothesis that β-lipotropin is the precursor or prohormone of the endogenous morphine-like peptides of pituitary origin. They also pointed out that the new peptides from both sheep and humans contain met-enkephalin, which was thought to be the active core.

Earlier in 1976, the isolation of the same 31-amino acid peptide from camel pituitary glands (74) and then human pituitary glands (75) had been reported. Their amino acid sequence was proposed to be identical to the sequence of the carboxyl-terminal 31 amino acids of human β-lipotropin, just as the factor isolated by Chretien et al. (20). The peptide reported by Li et al. (75) was designated β-endorphin and was shown to possess significant opiate activity in the guinea pig ileum. Similarly, Seidah et al. (113) replicated in part the results of Chretien et al. (20), reporting the complete amino acid sequence of the β-endorphin which had been isolated from the sheep pituitary. The sheep β-endorphin was identical to that of the portion 61-91 of sheep β-lipotropin (β-LPH).

Frederickson et al. (32) extracted material from human brain which had morphine-like activity on the mouse vas deferens. Bioassay and pharmacological activities were the same as porcine endorphin and enkephalin. Natural endorphins and enkephalins have been found in all mammals studied, including the camel, pig, cow, rat, mouse, guinea pig, and rabbit, as well as in human beings, and in other vertebrates, but not in invertebrates (114). This latter finding coincides with the reports on the discovery of opiate receptors in the brains of these subjects.

Distributions of the endorphin content of bovine pituitary and brain were determined by Queen et al. (105). The intermediate pituitary has 7, 15, 780, and 9100 times as much endorphin as the posterior pituitary, anterior pituitary, midbrain, and cortex, respectively. In pituitary, endorphins are localized to secretory granules common to all lobes. In the brain there is a similar granule, but it is derived at least in part from nerve endings. Using immunofluorescence methods, Bloom et al. (8) established the pituitary localizations of the endorphins to be in the pars intermedia (intermediate lobe) and the pars distalis (anterior lobe, adenophypophysis) of the pituitary, but not in the pars nervosa (posterior lobe, neurohypophysis) of the pituitary. LaBella et al. (72) also looked at endorphin concentrations in the pituitary and brain. The intermediate pituitary was the most concentrated.

Krieger et al. (69) published a report of the assays of discrete areas of bovine brain for β-LPH, adrenocorticotropin, and β-endorphin. β-endorphin concentrations showed marked variability within different portions of the limbic system, with the hypothalamus having the highest concentration, followed by the hippocampus. There was no correlation between the pattern of distribution of β-endorphin and β-LPH in the brain, although LaBella et al. (72) did report a parallel distribution for them in the pituitary. It was suggested that β-LPH may serve as a precursor of β-endorphin, since the higher concentrations of endorphin compared with β-LPH in the hypothalamus and hippocampus may reflect enzymatic degradation of β-LPH.

In order to determine the origin of the endorphins and enkephalins, Cheung and Goldstein (19) extracted endorphin-like activity from the brains of hypophysectomized rats and sham-operated controls on the 34th postoperative day. Since there was no significant difference in the opioid peptide content between the groups, the investigators concluded that the brain endorphin-like activity does not come from the pituitary, but is probably synthesized in the brain.

In addition to β-endorphin, two other forms of endorphin—α-endorphin and γ-endorphin—have been isolated from the porcine hypothalamic-pituitary extracts by Guillemin et al. (46). The primary structures of these endorphins correspond to sequences 61-76 of β-lipotropin for α-endorphin and 61-77 for γ-endorphin. These endorphins exhibited some opiate activity in the guinea pig ileum. Later Ling (77) reported the synthesis by solid-phase methodology of α-endorphin and γ-endorphin, which were shown to have the same physical, chemical, and opiate activity as the respective native substances. Marks et al. (81) reported that α-endorphin is much less potent than β-endorphin with in vivo measures, and the former does not produce the marked effects, such as immobility, that have been associated with β-endorphin (61), perhaps due, at least in part, to their differential rates of degradation. It is still not clear whether these two endorphins exist separately in the central nervous system (CNS) or are merely degradation products of β-endorphin.

Geisow and Smyth (35) found that the resistance of β-endorphin to the action of exopeptidases is due to consecutive lysine residues in the COOH-terminal sequence. These residues appear to be of importance with regard to the affinity of β-endorphin for the opiate receptors and, hence, for the potency of the peptide as an analgesic agent. A later study (34) indicated that a COOH-terminal tetrapeptide, Lys-Lys-Gly-Gln is also involved in the unique affinity of the β-endorphin for the opiate receptors. The presence of all four residues, not just the lysine ones, was found to be important for the high analgesic potency. The terminal region serves to confer stability on the peptide against proteolysis. Further support for this notion comes from the known instability of the enkephalins, which lack this terminal region.

CENTRAL NERVOUS SYSTEM EFFECTS

Just as the biochemical aspects of enkephalins and endorphins have been investigated, much research has also been done on their CNS correlates, both at the single-cell level and at a more molar level. Many researchers started by comparing the effects of morphine, which were fairly well established, with those of these new neuropeptides. Although the analgesic properties of the enkephalins and endorphins are some of their most striking and interesting characteristics, discussion of that aspect of the neuropeptides will be reserved for a later point in the chapter. Bradley et al. (13) applied met-enkephalin, morphine, or etorphine (a more potent analgesic than morphine) to single neurons of the rat brainstem. All three agents depressed activity of the cells, which was reversed by naloxone. Morphine and met-enkephalin also produced some excitation of the cells, which was not reversed by naloxone. Since the brainstem has been shown to be an important site for nociceptive action (6) and since the effects of enkephalin were similar to that of morphine, it might be suggested that enkephalin plays a role in pain perception. Bradley et al. (13) concluded that their findings supported the concept of a physiological role for endogenous enkephalin in the CNS, but whether that role involved pain perception remained an open question. The depressant action was thought to be more important physiologically than the excitatory one, since the depressant action alone was naloxone reversible.

In a similar study, Gent and Wolstencroft (36) studied the effects of met-enkephalin and leu-enkephalin in comparison with those of morphine on the brainstem neurons of the cat. Both enkephalins had inhibitory actions similar to those of morphine. Of particular interest were the effects on the reticular neurons, since they respond to noxious stimulation (16). Strong inhibition was noted for all three agents tested, suggesting a possible role in pain suppression. A surprising finding in this study was that none of these effects were blocked by naloxone. The authors concluded that the receptors responsible for these inhibitory actions in the cat brainstem must be different from those in rat brainstem and in the peripheral system.

Hill et al. (52) extended the findings of Bradley et al. (13) and Gent and Wolenstencroft (36) to include other areas of the brain, some of which are activated by painful stimuli, by taking recordings from the cerebral cortex, thalamus, and dorsal medulla. Met-enkephalin depressed the action of these neurons, including those in the thalamus which had previously fired in response to noxious stimulation, suggesting to the authors that enkephalin may be important as an inhibitory transmitter at both nociceptive and other sites. Data from a study by Frederickson and Norris (31) are also compatible with this notion of an neurotransmitter or neuromodulator role for enkephalin. They found that enkephalin and morphine depressed the firing of single neurons in the frontal cortex, caudate nucleus, and the periaqueductal gray matter, where enkephalin and a high concentration of opiate receptors are found.

Zieglgansberger et al. (135) described the effects of the application of synthetic enkephalin on the cortical neurons of naive and morphine-dependent rats. The enkephalin decreased the firing rate and was naloxone reversible in the naive rats. Inhibition was abolished in the morphine-dependent rats. Since these effects parallel those with morphine, it was concluded that enkephalin may have tolerance/dependence properties, too.

Since the guinea pig ileum has been shown to contain high concentrations of enkephalins (117), North and Williams (89) applied enkephalin to the myenteric plexus of the guinea pig ileum to investigate its action. Previous work (92) had shown that narcotic analgesics inhibit the electrically stimulated neuronal firing in this preparation. Low concentrations of enkephalins also inhibited their firings, with met-enkephalin being about five times as potent as leu-enkephalin and five to ten times more potent than morphine. Enkephalin was less potent on the longitudinal muscle strip than on isolated ganglia, presumably because a large portion of the dose for the former was bound nonspecifically and subsequently destroyed by peptidase. Since the inhibition was reversed by naloxone, the investigators concluded that the enkephalin was acting on the opiate receptors. The exact nature of the mechanism of the inhibition was not determined, so this study contributed no direct evidence concerning the question of the neurotransmitter role of enkephalins.

Urca et al. (128) studied the effects of intracerebroventricular (ICV) administration of doses of morphine and met-enkephalin on the multiple unit activity of the periaqueductal gray matter of the awake rat. While the morphine produced analgesia and increased multiple unit firing, only 8 of 19 rats showed analgesia with the met-enkephalin. However, in all 8 of them, and in no others, increased multiple unit activity was also seen, suggesting a strong relationship between the neural activity studied and analgesia. These findings supported the view that the periaqueductal gray matter is actively involved in endogenous mechanisms of pain reduction. An interesting observation also noted was that enkephalin caused electrographic and behavioral epileptic phenomena in most animals. This observation suggested to the investigators that enkephalin may play some as yet undetermined role in epileptogenesis. Audiogenic seizures, on the other hand, were decreased by injections of met-enkephalin into mice (100). This latter phenomenon was thought to be related in part to changes in brain concentrations of dihydroxyphenylalanine (DOPA), which was found to be potentiated by the enkephalin and which has been shown to modulate audiogenic seizures (63).

Using a different approach to test the hypothesized neurotransmitter role of endorphins, Puig et al. (104) produced electrically induced contractions of the myenteric plexus-longitudinal muscle preparation of the guinea pig ileum. A marked inhibition of the contractions appeared after the stimulation and this inhibition was reversed by several opiate antagonists. These findings suggested that the opiate receptors of the myenteric plexus had been activated due to the release of endogenous endorphins in response to the electrical stimulation. Thus, Puig et al. felt that they had demonstrated that endorphins have an inhibitory effect on at least some neuronal pathways.

On the other hand, Goldstein et al. (43) reported no support for the hypothesis that an endogenous opioid modulates responsiveness to pain and discomfort, since rats treated with doses of naloxone sufficient to block morphine analgesia showed no change in the threshold for escape from foot shock. If aversive stimuli resulted in the activation of opiate receptors by enkephalin or endorphin, the investigators reasoned that it should follow that blocking the receptors with naloxone should lower the shock escape threshold. Since naloxone produced no effect, it was concluded that endogenous opioids had not been produced, although it is possible that sensory discrimination of the stimulus, rather than the pain per se, maintained the escape response, thus making pain perception irrelevant to the response.

In the first of the few studies dealing with the effects of enkephalin on learning, Kastin et al. (65) administered met-enkephalin, a potent opiate analog [D-Ala^2]-Met-enkephalin-NH$_2$, a weak opiate analog [D-Phe^4]-Met-enkephalin, and morphine to hungry rats to test maze learning for food reward. Both the enkephalin and its analogs produced faster running and fewer errors than the diluent controls. The morphine-injected rats appeared to run slower and had more errors than the controls. Controls for appetite, thirst, olfaction, and general activity effects were tested, with the finding that none of these variables appeared responsible for the differences found. Kastin et al. concluded that enkephalin and some of its analogs exert significant changes in behavior, independent of opiate effects.

Michell et al. (85) also investigated learning effects in goldfish related to enkephalin and endorphin analogs—[D-Ala^2]-Met-enkephalin and [D-Ala^2]-β-endorphin—using a habituation task. The endorphin analog produced significantly longer latencies than the other two groups, which were not different from one another, although the investigators concluded that the effect was probably due to an immobilization reaction caused by the endorphin analog rather than by a learning mechanism per se.

The immobilization reported by Michell et al. (85) had been demonstrated in rats previously. Simultaneously, Bloom et al. (9) and Jacquet and Marks (61) published studies of immobility produced by β-endorphin and reversed by naloxone. Bloom et al. found a marked, prolonged muscular rigidity and immobility, similar to a catatonic state, lasting for hours in rats injected with β-endorphin, but not with met-enkephalin, α-endorphin, or γ-endorphin. The last three did, however, evoke dose-related, naloxone-reversible wet-dog shakes, as did the stronger β-endorphin. These potent and divergent responses to naturally occurring substances suggested that alterations in their homeostatic regulation could have etiological significance in mental illness.

Jacquet and Marks (61) noted similar reactions, with profound sedation and catalepsy resulting from injection of β-endorphin into the periaqueductal gray of the rat brain. Reflexes were diminished, analgesia was produced, animals remained immobile, and although able to move when startled, the affect was blunted, with many rats exhibiting the waxy-flexibility characteristic of catatonic states. Small fragments of met-enkephalin, leu-enkephalin, and α-endorphin produced attenuated forms of this behavior, but only at high dose levels, whereas β-endorphin produced it with only moderate doses. Jacquet and Marks concluded that β-endorphin is an important neuro-modulator of the CNS and suggested that it may play an etiological role in some psychopathological states, although the mechanism differed from that of Bloom et al. (9).

A later study by Segal et al. (112), however, suggested that β-endorphin is probably not a neuroleptic or antipsychotic agent, since it produced different behavioral reactions than haloperidol, a known neuroleptic. Segal et al. injected β-endorphin into the rat periaqueductal gray matter and observed rigid immobility and loss of the righting reflex. Rigidity was preceded or followed by hyperactivity, depending on the dose level. Haloperidol did not produce these behaviors at any dose, and produced stationary behavior when tested on a vertical grid, while β-endorphin produced sliding off or climbing off. These vast behavioral differences suggested that β-endorphin cannot be considered a neuroleptic.

Izumi et al. (58) also reported that ICV administration of β-endorphin in the rat produced akinesia or catalepsy and loss of the corneal reflex. Apomorphine injection reversed the akinesia, while pretreatment with α-methyl-p-tyrosine potentiated muscle rigidity. The behavioral findings were related to biochemical analysis of parts of the brains of rats injected with β-endorphin, leading to the conclusion that dopaminergic neurons are involved in the action of β-endorphin. There had been earlier suggestions of the involvement of the dopaminergic system by Plotnikoff et al. (106) in the first demonstration of a peripheral action of enkephalin.

A further demonstration of the immobilization response was noted by Olson, Olson, Wolf, Kastin, and Coy in an unpublished observation. Squirrel monkeys were injected with large doses of [D-Ala^2]-β-endorphin through a spinal tap. Sedation, profound analgesia, rigidity, uncoordination of fine movements, and immobility were reported. In addition, lack of pupillary response and lack of righting response, as well as some waxy-flexibility and resemblance of wet-dog shakes were also noted. The effects lasted approximately 4 hr. A smaller dose, injected peripherally, produced no noticeable behavioral changes at all. The relative importance of injection site, dose level, and blood-brain barrier has not yet been determined.

As previously noted, one of the approaches to the study of the behavioral effects of the opiate-like neuropeptides was to compare the effects of morphine and the enkephalins and endorphins. One of the classic features of opiates is the tolerance/dependence phenomenon. It was originally hoped that the new peptides would produce the beneficial effects of morphine, like analgesia, without the development of tolerance and dependence, since the peptides were naturally occurring substances. However, this hope does not seem to have been fulfilled.

Szekely et al. (120) performed experiments to establish the development of cross tolerance between morphine and β-endorphin in rats. Repeated ICV or peripheral administration of morphine induced tolerance both to morphine and β-endorphin. The tolerance induced by ICV administration of morphine was more pronounced than that produced by peripheral administration. The results led the investigators to conclude that, at least in part, similar sites and mechanisms are involved in the analgesic activity of morphine and endorphins. In a similar manner, Waterfield et al. (133) studied the interaction between enkephalin and morphine. They showed the development of cross tolerance between morphine and met-enkephalin occurring in the guinea pig ileum and in the mouse vas deferens when the animals had been implanted with morphine tablets. Thus, both enkephalin and endorphin have been shown to develop cross tolerance with the exogenous opiate, morphine.

Wei and Loh (134) infused met-enkephalin and β-endorphin for 70 hr into the periaqueductal gray and fourth ventricular spaces of the rat brain. Naloxone then was administered, producing typical morphine-like withdrawal symptoms. Thus, it was concluded that the natural peptides, like the exogenous agents, caused physical dependence by their presence in constant or higher than normal levels.

However, Fratta et al. (30) found no change in the level of met-enkephalin in the brain after withdrawal of morphine from dependent rats or after foot-shock stress. The failure to find an increase in enkephalin content after foot-shock stress was in contrast with reports of Madden et al. (79) and Rossier et al. (110). Differences in the results of Fratta et al. and previous research might have been due to different methodologies. In addition, Fratta et al. pointed out that there may have been an increase in β-endorphin, but they measured only met-enkephalin and so had no data on the former. The study of Rossier et al. (110) can shed further light on the subject, since β-endorphin was shown to be released from the pituitary during foot-shock induced stress with up to a sixfold increase in the plasma. However, the released β-endorphin did not accumulate in the brain. On the contrary, hypothalamic levels of β-endorphin were slightly, but significantly, reduced after the stress. Since Fratta et al., however, measured only met-enkephalin in the brain, the results of the two studies are not, in fact, contradictory at all.

A mechanism for the development of tolerance and dependence for exogenous opiates involving changes in the production of the endogenous opiate-like peptides was proposed by Kosterlitz and Hughes (68). They suggested that enkephalins or endorphins are normally involved as part of an inhibitory mechanism for transmitter release. With the use of morphine, however, the body becomes dependent on the exogenous agent to perform the neural inhibition function to the extent that the body does not produce its own opioid substances. Since there is this decrease in production of enkephalins or endorphins, more morphine is needed to replace them and still less endogenous material is produced. When morphine is discontinued, the body is temporarily left with no inhibitory mechanism at all and the withdrawal syndrome results. The development of cross tolerance between morphine and enkephalin or endorphin mentioned earlier (120, 133) supports the notion of the interaction between endogenous and exogenous opiate-like agents. Further support for this hypothesis of tolerance and dependence came from the study of Wei and Loh (134) in which the natural production of enkephalin and endorphin by the body might have ceased due to the constant presence of the infused peptides in the brain, making natural production unnecessary.

Although the study of Fratta et al. (30) seems to contradict this hypothesis, since no change in the level of enkephalin was found after morphine dependence, such might not be the case after all. It could be, as the investigators suggested, that the content of β-endorphin or the synthesis and release of enkephalins which was not measured might have significantly decreased, resulting in the dependence on morphine. There is no evidence at this point relating to the possible interaction of enkephalin and endorphin concerning this mechanism.

Another behavior which has been associated with morphine injections in rats is grooming (39). Excessive grooming in rats induced by α- and β-endorphin, as well as ACTH, β-MSH, LPH$_{61-69}$, and morphine, has also been demonstrated after ICV administration (40). Morphine and β-endorphin were equally potent and were more potent than the other substances; the grooming effects of both were reversed by naloxone. Leu- and met-enkephalin did not produce any grooming behavior at all. More recent results also show that β-endorphin can induce grooming after peripheral injection (129). Although the significance of these findings is unclear, they reinforce the possibility that there might be other physiological effects, perhaps even more important than the analgesic activity, of these neuropeptides.

Pert and Sivit (93) reported the hyperactivity of rats who had been injected with morphine, [D-Ala^2] met-enkephalinamide, or apomorphine. The rats were injected in the nucleus accumbens in the limbic forebrain, since that area has been shown to play a role in motility (66) and to contain opiate receptors (98). All three agents produced hyperactivity, with morphine and the enkephalin analog having a gradual onset, but with morphine lasting longer. The apomorphine produced an immediate increase in both horizontal and vertical spontaneous activity. Pert and Sivit suggested the existence in the brain of a tonically active enkephalinergic system with a role in modulating some aspects of motor activity.

Bergmann et al. (7) administered met-enkephalin or leu-enkephalin in the ventral thalamus or the lateral ventricle of rats. Only weak signs of the stereotyped behavior produced by morphine were observed. The stage of biting and gnawing was not reached, presumably because the enkephalins were degraded before the behavioral syndrome reached that stage. Interestingly, Belluzzi and Stein (5) noted that enkephalins may share not only the analgesic but also the euphorigenic properties of morphine, since they found that rats will work for enkephalin injection delivered into the lateral ventricle of the brain. Rates of bar pressing were higher for enkephalin and morphine than for Ringer's solution or a structurally similar but nonopiate peptide. Surprisingly, preference for leu-enkephalin was stronger than for met-enkephalin and about equivalent to that of morphine, although with other measures, met-enkephalin appears to be more potent. Belluzzi and Stein speculated that leu-enkephalin may be a natural reward transmitter or euphorigen. This notion is further supported by findings that areas that produce high rates of self-stimulation (37) overlap with areas known to contain enkephalin (29).

Some reasearchers, upon seeing the dramatic immobilization effects of β-endorphin reported by Bloom et al. (9) and Jacquet and Marks (61), tested the hypothesis suggested in both of those studies, that β-endorphin is related in some way to psychopathic states in the individual. Kline et al. (67) injected synthetic β-endorphin into three schizophrenic and two depressed patients. Schizophrenics experienced increased cognitive difficulties, while the depressed patients showed improvement on the first testing. A second testing produced no significant effects, while a third testing produced improvement in schizophrenics, especially after antipsychotic medication had been discontinued.

Since β-endorphin produced the marked catatonic states and since naloxone is known to reverse the effects of β-endorphin, it seems logical that naloxone might have some effect on schizophrenic behavior. Support for that notion came from Terenius et al. (124), who reported that levels of β-endorphin-like material are elevated in the cerebrospinal fluid of schizophrenics and that these levels return to normal when the patients improve clinically. If the level of β-endorphin can be reduced or if it can be made ineffective by an antagonist, perhaps the behavior would improve concomitantly. Gunne et al. (48) did, indeed, find reduction of schizophrenic hallucinations with injections of naloxone. But Volavka et al. (130) could not replicate those results, finding no improvement in the patient's hallucinatory behavior with naloxone treatments. Thus, the role of endorphins in the etiology of schizophrenia remains unsettled.

NEUROHUMORAL INTERACTIONS

Not surprisingly, enkephalins and endorphins have also been shown to interact with and to affect the production and distribution of biogenic amines. Some of these interactions may give us clues concerning the physiological function of the neuropeptides. The notion that they may play a role as a neuromodulator or neurotransmitter is supported by evidence that enkephalin and endorphin interact with dopamine. Plotnikoff et al. (100) found that met-enkephalin markedly potentiated the behavioral effects of d,1-DOPA when injected into mice. The effects were less with morphine, but even more striking with [D-Ala^2]-met-enkephalin, persisting at least 2 hr. The effect of enkephalin in the serotonin-potentiation test was minimal and the investigators suggested that the effects may involve dopaminergic receptor mechanisms. Loh et al. (78) found almost complete inhibitions of striatal dopamine release from the CNS with injections of β-endorphin. β-endorphin was twice as potent as morphine, while met-enkephalin was much less effective. Thus, clearly there is an interaction between a known neurotransmitter, dopamine, and the new opiate-like neuropeptides.

Acetylcholine production in the body has also been shown to be influenced by enkephalin and endorphin. Moroni et al. (87) found that analgesic doses of β-endorphin injected ICV decreased acetylcholine turnover rate in the cortex, hippocampus, nucleus accumbens, and globus pallidus, but not in the nucleus caudatus. Morphine also decreased the turnover rate. The effects of both were naloxone reversible. However α-endorphin failed to cause analgesia or to decrease acetylcholine turnover rate in all the brain nuclei studied. The decrease in the turnover rate produces a decrease in the firing rate to the neurons. In addition, natural enkephalins were shown by Jhamandos et al. (62) to interact with the opiate receptors in the brain to modulate the release of acetylcholine from the cholinergic neurons. Both met- and leu-enkephalin produced inhibition of acetylcholine release in vivo in rats, which was completely blocked by naloxone.

Goldstein et al. (41) reported endorphin has the typical opioid effect of inhibiting the adenylate cyclase activity of neuroblastoma X glioma NG 108-15 homogenates. The effects of endorphin were 10 to 100 times as potent as those of morphine, depending on the measure used, and both were naloxone reversed. The investigators suggested that the findings may relate to a possible physiological function of endorphins in the nervous system.

Gero (38) studied the effects of enkephalins on human serum esterase. Opioid agonists are known to accelerate the hydrolytic action of serum esterase, while antagonists competitively reverse this acceleration. Met-enkephalin had no activity, neither accelerating nor competing with an opioid accelerator. As a result, Gero proposed that met-enkephalin is only a prosthetic group of the true endogenous morphine-like factor and is too short a peptide chain to have a stable enough structure for opioid action in the presence of dissolved protein. This finding is in harmony with the absence of anything but weak analgesia being reported with peripheral administration (4), as will be discussed later, but may not be pertinent for nonopiate changes (65).

Hormones and their production have also been shown to be affected by enkephalins and endorphins. Guillemin et al. (47) demonstrated that β-endorphin and adrenocorticotropin (ACTH) are concomitantly secreted in increased amounts by the adenohypophysis in response to acute stress or adrenalectomy. A purifed corticotropin-releasing factor and other secret-agogues also elicit their secretion in vitro, while the administration of the synthetic glucocorticoid dexamethasone inhibits the secretion of both ACTH and β-endorphin. Thus, both substances seem to possess common and identical regulatory mechanisms, suggesting that there may be a functional role for circulating β-endorphin other than an opiate-like function.

Prolactin has also been shown to be affected by met- and leu-enkephalin after administration to rats (76). Met-enkephalin produced a consistent increase in plasma prolactin, while leu-enkephalin produced variable results. Both enkephalins released prolactin in monolayer cell cultures of rat pituitaries. Cocchi et al. (21) also studied the effects of leu-enkephalin and morphine on prolactin release and on growth hormone release. They found that leu-enkephalin stimulates the release of both hormones, as does morphine. They reported that the release of growth hormone by leu-enkephalin, but not that of prolactin by leu-enkephalin, involves specific opiate receptors, whereas the morphine release of both of the two hormones is through specific opiate receptors.

Cusan et al. (25) tested met-enkephalin, β-endorphin, and two analogs, [D-Ala^2]-met-enkephalin and [D-Ala^2]-met-enkephalinamide, for their prolactin and growth hormone-releasing activity. They found that met-enkephalin led to the stimulation of both prolactin and growth hormone release and that β-endorphin and the two analogs were 500–2000 times more potent in stimulating the release of the hormones. The differences in activity were assumed to be due to rapid deactivation of met-enkephalin. Dupont et al. (27) also tested β-endorphin and met-enkephalin for their ability to release prolactin. A 0.5 μg dose of β-endorphin injected intravenously (iv) produced a sevenfold increase in prolactin release, while 500 μg of met-enkephalin produced a fourfold increase. Both agents had more potent and rapid stimulatory effect after intracerebral injection. Dupont et al. suggested that enkephalin may act endogenously to control prolactin secretion through inhibition of dopamine release in median eminence, whereas growth hormone secretion may be controlled through release of growth hormone-releasing hormone from the hypothalamus.

ANALGESIA

Finally we come to one of the most striking and frequently studied characteristics of the enkephalins and endorphins, their ability to produce analgesia. The findings in this area have significant theoretical implications regarding the possible physiological roles of these neuropeptides and the perception of pain. Studies before the discovery of the existence of opiate peptides had reported that electrical stimulation of the brain resulted in analgesia. Reynolds (107) demonstrated that electrical stimulation in the dorsolateral perimeter of the midbrain central gray produced analgesia for exploratory survey of the brain. Termination of stimulation produced responsiveness to aversive stimuli, thus confirming that it was the electrical stimulation that produced the analgesic effects. Mayer et al. (82) reported that electrical stimulation at several mesencephalic and diencephalic sites inhibited responses to intense pain in rats while leaving responses to other sensory modes relatively unaffected.

Akil and Mayer (2) found that analgesia produced by electrical stimulation, like that produced by morphine, may depend on the integrity of serotonergic transmission, since p-CPA, a serotonin inhibitor, disrupted the analgesic response. Naloxone was also found to partially reverse the analgesia produced by electrical stimulation (3), suggesting the possibility that this analgesia may result, in part, from the release of endogenous opiate-like substances, such as enkephalins or endorphins. Hosobuchi et al. (54) also demonstrated pain relief by electrical stimulation of the central gray matter in human beings and its reversal by naloxone.

Pomeranz and Chiu (103) found that electroacupuncture in awake mice produced analgesia to noxious heat. Naloxone completely abolished it, implicating endorphins and/or enkephalins. Administration of naloxone to control mice produced hyperanalgesia, suggesting to the investigators that opiate peptides are released at a low basal rate in "normal" mice and at a much higher rate during acupuncture.

From these studies and with the knowledge that at least some of the areas which produced electrically stimulated analgesia contained opiate receptors, it seemed only logical to investigate further the analgesic properties of the enkephalins and endorphins. Belluzzi et al. (4) found that met-enkephalin and leu-enkephalin, when administered through permanently indwelling cannulae in lateral ventricles of rats, induced profound analgesia in vivo that was fully reversible by naloxone. Both enkephalins were less potent than morphine. It was suggested that these results supported the notion that enkephalin may serve as a natural opiate-like neurohormone in a central mechanism for the inhibition of pain, as proposed by Hughes (55).

Buscher et al. (15) compared the effects of morphine, met-enkephalin, and leu-enkephalin after ICV and iv administration in the mouse. Morphine was 75 and 240 times more active than met-enkephalin and leu-enkephalin, respectively, with the iv doses of the enkephalins producing only very short-acting and weak analgesia, in large part because of rapid degradation of the peptides. Naloxone blocked morphine and met-enkephalin, but, surprisingly, not leu-enkephalin. Malick and Goldstein (80) found that with intracerebral injections directly into the periaqueductal gray matter, however, met-enkephalin, leu-enkephalin, and morphine all produced potent, short-acting analgesic effects.

Ronai et al. (109) administered β-lipotropin and some of its fragments ICV to rats. β-Lipotropin produced analgesia 2.2 times weaker than morphine, while met-enkephalin and other fragments were completely ineffective. Naloxone reversed the effect of β-lipotropin. The investigators suggested that enzymatic cleavage occurs in the brain to produce the active forms of β-lipotropin. Graf et al. (44) also compared the analgesic effects of met-enkephalin and other lipotropin fragments that contain the complete structure of met-enkephalin at the NH_2 terminus. Their results showed that in vivo effects are a function of the length of the peptide chain, with met-enkephalin being the least potent and LPH_{61-91} peptide the most potent. The enkephalin effect was short-lasting (6-8 min), while the effects of morphine and the larger fragments had not even maximized by that time. The relative inefficiency and short duration of enkephalin was thought to be due to its rapid degradation by enzymes.

Contradictory results were reported by Leybin et al. (73), with ICV infusion of met-enkephalin producing increased, rather than decreased, responsiveness to noxious stimuli. In addition, the met-enkephalin also induced behavior typical of opiate withdrawal. Both morphine and leu-enkephalin produced the expected analgesic effects, so it is doubtful that the results were due to methodological irregularities. Instead, the authors suggested that the lack of the usual analgesic effect might be due to the inability of met-enkephalin to reach sites of opiate analgesic action in the caudal portions of the ventricular system due to rapid degradation of the peptide. Another explanation offered was the possibility that met-enkephalin might have excited sites of "paradoxical" opiate action, a response such as that found by Jacquet and Lathja (60), who reported paradoxical, concurrent hyperactivity and hyporeactivity to specific stimuli after injections of morphine in the periaqueductal gray of rats.

The possibility that the test conditions might have induced mobilization and release of a more potent endogeneous substance in the brain, which also acts on the opiate receptors, was suggested (73). This endogenous substance could have become adapted to within several minutes, producing tolerance and dependence. If, then, the weaker injected met-enkephalin displaced the more potent endogenous substance, the withdrawal symptoms noted would not be unexpected. They further suggested that leu-enkephalin and morphine did not produce these results because they are purer agonists than met-enkephalin. More data relevant to this hypothesis need to be gathered before one can adequately explain this unexpected lack of analgesia, however.

Analgesic effects of β-endorphin have been reported after iv injection (126). Pretreatment with naloxone eliminated the analgesia. β-Endorphin was 3 to 4 times as potent as morphine injected iv. Ree et al. (106) confirmed the analgesic potency of the β-endorphin when administered ICV to the rat. They also showed that chronic administration of the peptide produces development of tolerance to its analgesic properties. Some cross tolerance to morphine also developed. The authors suggested that the mechanisms involved in the production of tolerance may be important in regulating the actions of endogenous opiate peptides in vivo and that other neuropeptides may play some part in modulating these processes.

A strong and long-lasting analgesia was found by Bradbury et al. (12) after ICV infusion of β-endorphin in the rat. Its analgesic properties were compared with those of three synthetic derivatives of met-enkephalin which presumably had been stabilized against enzymatic degradation. β-endorphin was 50 times as potent as N-methyl met-enkephalin amide. Singly blocked peptides produced only transient analgesia. Analgesia seemed dependent on the length and nature of the peptide, not on its resistance to degradation.

Human β-endorphin was also found by Tseng et al. (127) to produce potent analgesia in rats with ICV administration. It was 21 times as potent as morphine, produced morphine-like catatonia and hyperthermia, and was blocked by naloxone. Repeated injections produced tolerance and cross tolerance to morphine was observed.

Walker et al. (131) reported that ICV administration of the enkephalin analog [D-Ala^2]-met-enkephalin induces profound and long-lasting analgesia and other opiate-like behavioral effects in the rat. This analgesia was highly dose-dependent, of much greater magnitude, and about 30 times longer lasting than that of met-enkephalin. Behavioral effects of the analog could be completely reversed by naloxone. Walker et al. (132) also looked at the analgesic effects of ICV administration of α-, γ-, and β-endorphin and their [D-Ala^2] analogs in the rat. Analgesia was produced by all substances. The actions of [D-Ala^2]-α-endorphin and [D-Ala^2]-β-endorphin were considerably greater than the parent forms, whereas [D-Ala^2]-γ-endorphin was approximately equivalent to its parent compound. All effects were naloxone reversible. It was suggested that these analogs might be useful in behavioral tests when a longer duration of action is desirable.

In a clinical study, Buchsbaum et al. (14) studied the effects of naloxone injection in normal subjects divided into pain-sensitive and pain-insensitive subgroups based on pretesting. The insensitive subjects found shocks significantly more painful after naloxone administration, while the sensitive group experienced them as less painful. These results suggested that individual differences in pain sensitivity may relate to differences in the brain opiates. They also suggested a modulatory rather than strictly analgesic role for endorphins.

RELATION TO PAIN

The fact that endorphins and enkephalins, as well as the exogenous opiate-like agents, produce analgesia, suggests that there is a possible physiological role for the endogenous substances in pain perception. Some of the evidence discussed in this chapter bears directly on this issue. One such line of support for this hypothesis is the fact that the distributions of the opiate receptors correspond in part to certain pathways in the nervous system that are known to be pain pathways (70) or to areas of the brain and brainstem thought to mediate pain (94). Since there is this close correspondence and since these receptors bind to agents known to reduce or remove pain, it seems reasonable to speculate that the receptors might function in some way to mediate pain perception. Since the opiate receptors are found mainly in nervous tissue (93), it is suggested that these receptors are related in some way to the transmission of pain impulses. It further follows logically that the endogenous ligands for these receptors could be responsible in some way for this regulation of pain. These ligands may well be enkephalins or endorphins, since Pasternak et al. (91) found the regional distribution of the enkephalins correlated with that of the opiate receptors and since administration of these neuropeptides does produce analgesia.

Another line of evidence suggesting the possible role of enkephalins or endorphins in the transmission of pain comes from a study of Terenius and Wahlstrom (122), in which they found that patients suffering from chronic pain from trigeminal neuralgia had a lower level of the MLF than normal individuals. Possibly the lowered level of the endogenous substance allowed the transmission of the pain or its central perception more readily. Terenius and Wahlstrom further noted that the level of MFL varied significantly among individuals, but they did not attempt to relate these differences to individual differences in sensitivity to pain. It would be interesting to test the correlation of these two variables to determine if there is a relationship existing between them.

Buchsbaum et al. (14) did attempt to relate individual differences in pain perception to differences in an endorphin system by studying the changes in pain sensitivity in both pain-sensitive and pain-insensitive subjects after injections of naloxone. Naloxone, being an opiate antagonist, presumably would act in a competitive fashion with endogenous enkephalins-endorphins. If these peptide opiates play any part in the regulation of pain, then naloxone administration, upon altering the availability of the enkephalins-endorphins to the receptors, should alter the perception of pain. A bidirectional function was observed, with some subjects increasing in sensitivity to a noxious stimulus and others decreasing, suggesting the possibility that enkephalins-endorphins may be functioning in pain perception, probably acting in a modulatory way, rather than strictly as a pain reducer. Supporting the notion of bidirectionality is the report of Leybin et al. (73) that met-enkephalin unexpectedly increased sensitivity to pain in rats. Buchsbaum et al. suggested that bidirectionality effects may reflect individual differences in the functional activity of the pain modulation systems.

It has also been shown that there is an increase in brain or circulating enkephalin or endorphin levels after foot shock (79, 110). If these neuropeptides are being released in response to painful stimulation, then they might be playing some kind of role in the transmission of the pain impulses, perhaps having the function of preparing the organism for pain or reducing further pain once it has initially been perceived.

Recordings from single cells that have been exposed to enkephalins or endorphins further suggest the possibility of a physiological role for these substances in the perception of pain. Since readings from areas known to be important sites for reception of noxious stimulation show naloxone-reversible decreased activity after administration of enkephalin or endorphin (e.g., refs 13, 36, 52), it might be suggested that the endogenous peptides have a similar physiological role in the inhibition of the firing of these neurons.

The possible neurotransmitter or neuromodulator role of these neuropeptides was supported by studies showing that they affect the action of (100) or the release of (78) dopamine and of acetylcholine (87, 62). Since both dopamine and acetylcholine have neurotransmitter functions and since they both interact with enkephalins and endorphins, it could be speculated that these peptides have a regulator role of some kind in the nervous system. The nature of that role, however, has yet to be determined, if indeed there is such a physiological function for the peptides.

Although many studies suggest that opiate analgesia occurs in the brain, Synder (119) noted that there is also a good deal of evidence indicating that at least some component of the analgesia takes place at the level of the spinal cord. If this is the case, it is conceivable that the opiate peptides might provide a central control mechanism affecting the opening or closing of the "gate" for pain perception according to the gate control theory originally proposed by Melzack and Wall (84). They suggested that there are inhibitory cells in the substantia gelatinosa which respond differentially to input from C (small) fibers and A (large) fibers to regulate the transmission of the pain impulse. The small fibers inhibit the cells, thus releasing the cells' inhibitory effect and permitting transmission of the impulse. The opposite action was thought to occur with large fibers, which excite the cells to provide their inhibitory action.

There is considerable disagreement about the evidence supporting this theory, with some workers unable to reproduce the disinhibition effect attributed to small fibers (e.g., refs 118, 88). Others, however, have demonstrated the existence of cells specifically responsive to C-fiber stimulation (71) and different cells whose basic response was either inhibition or excitation in response to noxious stimulation (17). Hentall (51) found a third type of cell in the substantia gelatinosa whose action is excited by C fibers and inhibited by A fibers, thus further supporting the idea that the substantia gelatinosa plays a role in pain transmission.

The gate theory has now undergone some revision, with more central control over the action of the substantia gelatinosa being postulated (83). Dykes (28) pointed out, however, that the theory is still inadequate because it does not resolve the problem of conflicting data and because it is incomplete in that it cannot account for analgesia produced by acupuncture or electrical stimulation. In answer to the second criticism, Pomeranz et al. (102) suggested that acupuncture analgesia may be mediated by morphine-like hormones or peptides released by the pituitary. They found that acupuncture reduced responses in the spinal cord neurons to noxious stimuli in both cats and mice, with analgesia prolonged after termination of the acupuncture stimulation. Analgesia was not found in hypophysectomized mice, implicating pituitary involvement in the analgesia. Further support for the role of pituitary substances in acupuncture analgesia was reported by O'Connor and Bensky (90) in cross-circulation experiments in rats in which the recipients experienced analgesia from acupuncture of the donor animals. The involvement of morphine-like substances in acupuncture was suggested by the demonstration that naloxone blocked acupuncture analgesia (163). It is possible that acupuncture analgesia involves the action of the opiate-like neuropeptides on the substantia gelatinosa of the spinal cord.

Duggan et al. (26) measured the responses of neurons of spinal laminae IV and V to stimulation of a digital pad by painful heat after injections of morphine, met-enkephalin, and met-enkephalin amide into the substantia gelatinosa of cats. These neurons had fired to the noxious heat stimulus prior to the injections. Morphine depressed the cell responses to the noxious stimulus, thus producing analgesia. The enkephalins also inhibited the firing of the cells, but in a less systematic fashion than did the morphine. Met-enkephalin amide inhibited 10 of the 11 cells tested, while met-enkephalin inhibited only 2 of the 6 tested. In addition, the effects of the enkephalins rapidly disappeared, with recovery being complete within 10 min of the termination of the injection.

Thus, it may possibly be that a physiological role of the enkephalins involves the partial or complete control of the spinal transmission of pain. Support for the speculation comes from the fact that there are opiate receptors in the substantia gelatinosa which apparently bound the morphine and the enkephalins in the study of Duggan et al. (26). It is possible that these receptors and their endogenous ligands function regularly in the control of pain perception. The precise mechanisms involved and their specific functional relevance to the pain fibers remain to be investigated. Nevertheless, a possible role in the peripheral transmission of pain is suggested for the opiate peptides.

Snyder (119) pointed out that, although the analgesia mediated at the spinal cord level must be presynaptic in nature, there is also evidence that in some parts of the brain opiates and enkephalins inhibit cell firings (e.g., ref. 135). These latter effects are postsynaptic. Thus, it is likely that opiates and endogenous opiate-like neuropeptides act on both postsynaptic and presynaptic opiate receptors in the spinal cord and brain. Guillemin (45) suggested that the same substance may be used as a neurotransmitter in one instance, a modulator in another, and a hormone in still another situation. The opioid neuropeptides may turn out to fit these characteristics, judging from the multiplicity of effects they seem to produce. Much research still remains to be done to determine the action or actions of the enkephalins and endorphins.

REFERENCES

1. Agarwal, N., Hruby, V., Katz, R., Klee, W., and Nirenberg, M. Synthesis of leucine enkephalin derivatives: Structure-function studies. *Biochem. Biophys. Res. Commun.* 76, 129-135 (1977).

2. Akil, H. and Mayer, D. Antagonism of stimulation-produced analgesia by p-CPA, a serotonin synthesis inhibitor. *Brain Res.* 44, 692-697 (1972).

3. Akil, H., Mayer, D.J., and Liebeskind, J.C. Antagonism of stimulation-produced analgesia by naloxone, a narcotic antagonist. *Science* 191, 961-962 (1976).

4. Belluzzi, J., Grant, N., Garsky V., Sarantakis, D., Wise, C., and Stein, L. Analgesia induced in vivo by central administration of enkephalin in rat. *Nature* 260, 625-626 (1976).

5. Belluzzi, J. and Stein, L. Enkephalin may mediate euphoria and drive-reduction reward. *Nature* 266, 556-558 (1977).

6. Benjamin, R.M. Single neurons in the rat medulla responsive to nociceptive stimulation. *Brain Res.* 24, 525-529 (1970).

7. Bergmann, F., Altstetter, R., Pasternak, V., Chaimovitz, M., Oreg, M., Roth, D., Hexter, C., and Wilchek, M. Cerebral application of enkephalins. *Experimentia* 217 (1977).

8. Bloom, F., Battenberg, E., Rossier, J., Ling, N., Leppaluoto, J., Vargo, T., and Guillemin, R. Endorphins are located in the intermediate and anterior lobes of the pituitary gland, not in the neurophypophysis. *Life Sci.* 20, 43-48 (1977).

9. Bloom, B., Segal, D., and Guillemin, R. Endorphins: Profound behavioral effects in rats suggest new etiological factors in mental illness. *Science* 194, 630-632 (1976).

10. Bradbury, A.F., Smyth, D.G., and Snell, C.R. Biosynthesis of β-MSH and ACTH. In *Peptides, Chemistry, Structure and Biology.* R. Walter and G. Meienhofer, ed. Ann Arbor Science, Mich., 1975, pp. 609-615.

11. Bradbury, D., Smyth, D., and Snell, C. Biosynthetic origin and receptor conformation of methionine and enkephalin. *Nature* 260, 165-166 (1976).

12. Bradbury, A., Smyth, D., Snell, C., Deakin, J., and Wendlant, S. Comparison of the analgesic properties of lipotropin C-fragment and stabilized enkephalins in the rat. *Biochem. Biophys. Res. Commun.* 74, 478-754 (1977).

13. Bradley, P., Briggs, I., Gayton, R., and Lambert, L. Effects of microiontophoretically applied methionine-enkephalin on single neurones in rat brainstem. *Nature* 261, 426-427 (1976).

14. Buchsbaum, M.S., Davis, G.C., and Bunney, W.E., Jr. Naloxone alters pain perception and somatosensory evoked potentials in normal subjects. *Nature* 270, 620-622 (1977).

15. Buscher, H., Hill, R., Roemer, D., Cardinaux, F., Closse, A., Hauser, D., and Pless, J. Evidence for analgesic activity of enkephalin in the mouse. *Nature* 261, 423-425 (1976).

16. Casey, K.L. Somatosensory responses of bulbo reticular units in awake cat: Relation to escape-producing stimuli. *Science* 173, 77-80 (1971).

17. Cervero, F., Ensor, D.R., Iggo, A., and Molony, V. Activity from single neurones recorded in the substantia gelatinsa Rolandi of the cat. *J. Physiol. (London)* 169, 37P-39P (1977).

18. Chang, J—K., Fong, B., Pert, A., and Pert, C. Opiate receptor affinities and behavioral effects of enkephalin: Structure-activity relationship of ten synthetic peptide analogues. *Life Sci.* 18, 1473-1482 (1976).

19. Cheung, A. and Goldstein, A. Failure of hypophysectomy to alter brain content of opioid peptides (endorphins). *Life Sci.* 19, 1005-1008 (1976).

20. Chretien, M., Benjannet, S., Dragon, N., Seidah, N., and Lis, M. Isolation of peptides with opiate activity from sheep and human pituitaries: Relationship to beta-lipotropin. *Biochemi. Biophys. Res. Commun.* 72, 472-478 (1976).

21. Cocchi, D., Santagostino, A., Gil-Ad, T., Ferri, S., and Muller, E. Leu-enkephalin-stimulated growth hormone and prolactin release in the rat: Comarison with the effect of morphine. *Life Sci.* 20, 2041-2046 (1977).

22. Cowie, A., Kosterlitz, H., and Watt, A. Mode of action of morphine-like drugs on automatic neuro-effectors. *Nature* 220, 1040-1042 (1968).

23. Coy, D., Kastin, A., Schally, A., Morin, O., Caron, N., Labrie, F., Walker, J., Fertel, R.,

Bernston, G., and Sandman, C. Synthesis and opioid activities of stereoisomers and other D-amino acid analogs of methionine-enkephalin. *Biochem. Biophyl. Res. Commun.* 73, 632-638 (1976).

24. Creese, I. and Snyder, S. Receptor binding and pharmacological activity of opiates in the guinea-pig intestine. *J. Pharmacol. Exp. Thera.* 194, 205-219 (1976).

25. Cusan, L., Dupont, A., Kledzik, G., Labrie, F., Coy, D., and Schally, A. Potent prolactin and growth hormone releasing activity of more analogues of met-enkephalin. *Nature* 268, 544-547 (1977).

26. Duggan, A., Davies, J., and Hall, J. Effects of opiate agonists and antagonists on central neurons of the cat. *J. Pharmacol. Exp. Thera.* 196, 107-120 (1976).

27. Dupont, A., Cusan, L., Labrie, F., Coy, D., and Li, C. Stimulation of prolactin release in the rat by intraventricular injection of β-endorphin and methionine-enkephalin. *Biochem. Biophys. Res. Commun.* 75, 76-81 (1977).

28. Dykes, R.W. Nociception. *Brain Res.* 99, 229-245 (1975).

29. Elde, R., Hokfelt, T., Johannsson, O., and Terenius, L. Immunohistochemical studies using antibodies to leucine-enkephalin: Initial observation on the nervous system of the rat. *Neuroscience* 1, 349-351 (1976).

30. Fratta, W., Yang, H-Y., Hong, J., and Costa, E. Stability of met-enkephalin in brain structures of morphine-dependent or foot shock-stressed rats. *Nature* 268, 452-453 (1977).

31. Frederickson, R. and Norris, F. Enkephalin-induced depression of single neurons in brain areas with opiate receptors—Antagonism by naloxone. *Science* 194, 440-442 (1976).

32. Frederickson, R., Schirmer, E., Grinnan, E., Harrell, C., and Hewes, C. Human endorphin: Comparison with porcine endorphin, enkephalin and normorphine. *Life Sci.* 19, 1181-1190 (1976).

33. Garbay-Jaureguiberry, C., Roques, B., and Oberlin, R. Preferential conformation of the endogenous opiate-like pentapeptide in DMSO-D$_6$ solution, *Biochem. Biophys. Res. Commun.* 71, 558-565 (1976).

34. Geisow, M., Deakin, J., Dostrovsky, J., and Smyth, D. Analgesic activity of lipotropin C-fragment depends on carboxyl terminal tetrapeptide. *Nature* 269, 167-168 (1977).

35. Geisow, M. and Smyth, D. Lipotropin C-fragment has a COOH-terminal sequence with high intrinsic resistance to the action of exopeptidases. *Biochem. Biophys. Res. Commun.* 75, 625-629 (1977).

36. Gent, J. and Wolstencroft, J. Effects of methionine-enkephalin and leucine-enkephalin compared with those of morphine on brainstem neurones in cat. *Nature* 261, 426-427 (1976).

37. German, D.C. and Bowden, D.M. Catecholamine systems as the neural substrate for intracranial self-stimulation: A hypothesis. *Brain Res.* 73, 381 (1974).

38. Gero, A. Inactivity of enkephalin on human serum esterase. *Life Sci.* 19, 479-482 (1976).

39. Gispen, W.H. and Wiegant, V.M. Opiate antagonists suppress ACTH$_{1-24}$-induced excessive grooming in the rat. *Neuroscience Lett.* 2, 159-164 (1976).

40. Gispen, W., Wiegant, V., Bradbury, A., Hulme, E., Smyth, D., and Snell, C. Induction of excessive grooming in the rat by fragments of lipotropin. *Nature* 264, 794-795 (1976).

41. Goldstein, A., Cox, B., Klee, W., and Nirenberg, M. Endorphin from pituitary inhibits cyclic AMP formation in homogenates of neuroblastoma X glioma hybrid cells. *Nature* 265, 362-363 (1977).

42. Goldstein, A., Lowney, L.I., and Pal, B.K. Stereospecific and nonspecific interactions of the morphine congener levorphanol in subcellular fractions of mouse brain. *Proc. Nat. Acad. Sci. USA* 68, 1742-1747 (1971).

43. Goldstein, A., Pryor, G., Otis, L., and Larsen, F. On the role of endogenous opioid peptides: Failure of naloxone to influence shock escape threshold in the rat. *Life Sci.* 18, 599-604 (1976).

44. Graf, L., Szekely, J. Ronai, A., Dunai-Kovacs, Z., and Bajusz, S. Comparative study on analgesic effect of Met^5-enkephalin and related lipotropin fragments. *Nature* 263, 240-241 (1976).

45. Guillemin, R. Discussion, in, S. Reichlin, R.J. Baldessarini, and J.B. Martin, ed. *The Hypothalamus.* Raven Press, New York, 1978, p. 215.

46. Guillemin, R., Ling, N., and Burgus, R. Endorphines: Peptides of hypothalamic and neurohypophyseal origin. Isolation and molecular structure of alpha-endorphine. *C.R. Acad. Sci. Ser. D* 283, 783-785 (1976).

47. Guillemin, R., Vargo, T., Rossier, J., Minick, S., Ling, N., Rivier, C., Vale, W., and Bloom, F. β-endorphin and adrenocortico-tropin are secreted concomitantly by the pituitary gland. *Science* 197, 1367-1369 (1977).

48. Gunne, L. M., Lindstrom, L., and Terenius, L. Naloxone-induced reversal of schizophrenic hallucinations. *Neural Transmitters* 40, 13-19 (1977).

49. Hambrook, J., Morgan, B., Rance, M., and Smith, C. Mode of deactivation of the enkephalins by rat and human plasma and rat brain homogenates. *Nature* 262, 782-783 (1976).

50. Henderson, G., Hughes, J., and Kosterlitz, H.W. A new example of a morphine-sensitive neuro-effector junction; adrenergic transmission in the mouse vas deferens. *Br. J. Pharmacol.* 46, 764-766 (1972).

51. Hentall, I. A novel class of unit in the substantia gelatinosa of the spinal cat. *Exp. Neurol.* 57, 792-806 (1977).

52. Hill, R., Pepper, C., and Mitchell, J. Depression of nociceptive and other neurones in the brain by iontophorectically applied met-enkephalin. *Nature* 262, 604-606 (1976).

53. Horn, A. and Rodgers, J. Structural and conformational relationships between the enkephalins and the opiates. *Nature* 260, 795-797 (1976).

54. Hosobuchi, Y., Adams, J., and Linchitz, R. Pain relief by electrical stimulation of central gray matter in humans and its reversal by naloxone. *Science* 197, 183-186 (1977).

55. Hughes, J. Isolation of an endogenous compound from the brain with pharmacological properties similar to morphine. *Brain Res.* 88, 295-308 (1975).

56. Hughes, J., Smith, T.W., Kosterlitz, H.W., Fothergill, L.A., Morgan, B.A., and Morris, H.R. Identification of two related pentapeptides from the brain with potent opiate agonist activity. *Nature* 258, 577-579 (1975).

57. Hughes, J., Smith, T.W., Morgan, B.A., and Fothergill, L.A. Purification and properties of enkephalin—the possible endogenous ligand for the morphine receptor. *Life Sci.* 16, 1753-1758 (1975).

58. Izumi, K., Motomatsu, T., Chretien, M., Butterworth, R., Lis, M., Seidah, N., and Barbeau, A. β-endorphin induced akinesia in rats: Effect of apomorphine and α-methyl-p-tryosine and related modifications of dopamine turnover in the basal ganglia. *Life Sci* 20, 1149-1156 (1977).

59. Jacquet, Y.F., Klee, W.A., Rice, K.C., Iijima, I., and Minamikawa, J. Stereospecific and nonstereospecific effect of (+) and (–) -morphine: Evidence for a new class of receptors? *Science* 198, 842-845 (1977).

60. Jacquet, Y.F. and Lathja, A. Paradoxical effects after microinjection of morphine in the periaqueductal gray matter in the rat. *Science* 185, 1055-1057 (1974).

61. Jacquet, Y.F. and Marks, N. The C-fragment of β-lipotropin: An endogenous neuroleptic or antipsychotogen? *Science* 194, 632-635 (1976).

62. Jhamandos, K., Swaynok, J., and Sutak, M. Enkephalin effects on release of brain acetylcholine. *Nature* 269, 433-434 (1977).

63. Jobe, P.C., Picchioni, A.L., and Chin, L. Role of brain norepinephrine in audiogenic seizure in the rat. *Pharmacol. Exp. Ther.* 184, 1-10 (1973).

64. Jones, C., Garsky, V., and Gibbons, W. Molecular conformations of met-enkephalin: Comparison of the zwitterionic and cationic forms. *Biochem. Biophys. Res. Commun.* 76, 619-625 (1977).

65. Kastin, A., Scollan, E., King, M., Schally, A., and Coy, D. Enkephalin and a potent analog facilitate maze performance after intrapertioneal administration in rats. *Pharmacol. Biochem. Behav.* 5, 691-695 (1976).

66. Kelly, P.H., Seviour, P.W., and Iverson, S.D. Amphetamine and apomorphine responses in the rat following 6-OHDA lesions of the nucleus accumbens septi and corpus striatum. *Brain Res.* 94, 507-522 (1975).

67. Kline, N., Li, C., Lehmann, J., Lajtha, A., Laski, E., and Cooper, T. β-endorphin-induced changes in schizophrenic and depressed patients. *Arch. Gen. Psychiatry* 34, 1111-1113 (1977).

68. Kosterlitz, H.W. and Hughes, J. Some thoughts on the significance of enkephalin, the endogenous ligand. *Life Sci.* 17, 91-96 (1975).

69. Krieger, D., Liotta, A., Suda, T., Palkovits, M., and Brownstein, M. Presence of immunoassayable β-lipotropin in bovine brain and spinal cord: Lack of concordance with ACTH concentrations. *Biochem. Biophys. Res. Commun.* 76, 930-936 (1977).

70. Kuhar, M., Pert, C., and Snyder, S. Regional distribution of opiate receptor binding in monkey and human brain. *Nature* 245, 447-450 (1973).

71. Kumazawa, T. and Perl, E.R. Differential excitation of dorsal horn and substantia gelatinosa marginal neurones by primary afferent units with fine (A and C) fibres, in *Sensory Functions of the Skin.* Y. Zotterman, ed., Pergamon, Oxford, 1976, pp. 67-89.

72. LaBella, F., Queen, G., and Senyshyn, J. Lipotropin: Localization by radioimmunoassay of endorphin precursor in pituitary and brain. *Biochem. Biophys. Res. Commun.* 75, 350-357 (1977).

73. Leybin, L., Pinsky, C., LaBella, F., Havlicek, V., and Rezek, M. Intraventricular met[5]-enkephalin causes unexpected lowering of pain threshold and narcotic withdrawal signs in rats. *Nature* 264, 458-459 (1976).

74. Li, C.H. and Chung, D. Isolation and structure of an untriakontapeptide with opiate activity from camel pituitary glands. *Proc. Nat. Acad. Sci. USA* 73, 1145-1148 (1976).

75. Li, C., Chung, D., and Doneen, B. Isolation, characterization and opiate activity of β-endorphin from human pituitary glands. *Biochem. Biophys. Res. Commun.* 72, 1542-1547 (1976).

76. Lien, E., Fenichel, R., Garsky, V., Sarantakis, D., and Grant, N. Enkephalin-stimulated prolactin release. *Life Sci.* 19, 837-840 (1976).

77. Ling, N. Solid phase synthesis of porcine α-endorphin and γ-endorphin, two hypothalamic-pituitary peptides with opiate activity. *Biochem. Biophys. Res. Commun.* 74, 248-254 (1977).

78. Loh, H., Brase, D., Sampath-Khanna, S., Mar, J., Way, E., and Li, C. β-endorphin in vitro inhibition of striatal dopamine release. *Nature* 264, 567-568 (1976).

79. Madden, I.V.J., Akil, H., Patrick, R.L., and Barchas, I.D. Stress-induced parallel changes in central opioid levels and pain responsiveness in the rat. *Nature* 265, 358-360 (1977).

80. Malick, J. and Goldstein, J. Analgesic activity of enkephalins following intracerebral administration in the rat. *Life Sci.* 20, 827-832 (1977).

81. Marks, N., Grynbaum, A., and Neidle, A. On the degradations of enkephalins and endorphins by rat and mouse extracts. *Biochem. Biophys. Res. Commun.* 74, 1552-1559 (1977).

82. Mayer, D., Wolfe, T., Akil, H., Carder, B., and Liebeskind, J. Analgesia from electrical stimulation in the brainstem of the rat. *Science* 174, 1351-1354 (1971).

83. Melzack, R. *The Puzzle of Pain.* Penguin Books, Harmondsworth, England, 1973.

84. Melzack, R. and Wall, P.D. Pain mechanisms: A new theory. *Science* 150, 971-979 (1965).
85. Michell, G., Olson, R.D., Kastin, A.J., Olson, G.A., Montalbano, D., and Coy, D.H. Effects of an endogenous analog on the habituation of an innate fear response in goldfish. Presented before the Society for Neuroscience, Anaheim, 1977.
86. Morin, O., Caron, M., DeLean, A., Labrie, F. Binding of the opiate-like pentapeptide methionine-enkephalin to a particular fraction from the rat brain. *Biochem. Biophys. Res. Commun.* 73, 940-946 (1976).
87. Moroni, F., Cheney, D., and Costa, E. β-endorphin inhibits ACh turnover in nuclei of rat brain. *Nature* 267, 267-268 (1977).
88. Mountcastle, V.B. Pain and temperature sensibilities, in *Medical Physiology,* 13th ed. V.B. Mountcastle, ed. Mosby, St. Louis, 1974, ch. 11.
89. North, R. and Williams, J. Enkephalin inhibits firing of myenteric neurones. *Nature* 264, 460-461 (1976).
90. O'Connor, J. and Bensky, D. A summary of research concerning the effects of acupuncture. *Am. J. Chin. Med.* 3, 377-394 (1975).
91. Pasternak, G., Goodman, R., and Snyder, S. An endogenous morphine-like factor in mammalian brain. *Life Sci.* 16, 1765-1769 (1975).
92. Paton, W.D.M. The action of morphine and related substances on contraction and on acetylcholine output of coaxially stimulated guinea-pig ileum. *Br. J. Pharmacol.* 12, 119-127 (1957).
93. Pert, A. and Sivit, C. Neuroanatomical focus for morphine and enkephalin-induced hypermotility. *Nature* 265, 645-647 (1977).
94. Pert, A. and Yaksh, T. Sites of morphine induced analgesia in the primate brain: Relation to pain pathways. *Brain Res.* 80, 135-140 (1974).
95. Pert, C., Aposhian, D., and Snyder, S. Phylogenetic distribution of opiate receptor binding. *Brain Res.* 75, 356-361 (1974).
96. Pert, C., Bowie, D., Pert, A., Morell, J., and Gross, E. Agonist-antagonist properties of N-allyl-[D-Ala^2]-met-enkephalin. *Nature* 269, 73-75 (1977).
97. Pert, C., Pasternak, G., and Snyder, S. Opiate agonists and antagonists discriminated by receptor binding in brain. *Science* 182, 1359-1361 (1973).
98. Pert, C., Pert, A., Chang, J., and Fong, B. [D-Ala^2]-met-enkephalinamide: A potent, long-lasting synthetic pentapeptide analgesic. *Science* 194, 330-332 (1976).
99. Pert, C. and Snyder, S. Opiate receptor: Demonstration in nervous tissue. *Science* 179, 1011-1014 (1973).
100. Plotnikoff, N., Kastin, A., Coy, D., Christensen, C., Schally, A., and Sprites, M. Neuropharmacological actions of enkephalins after systematic administration. *Life Sci.* 19, 1283-1287 (1976).
101. Pollard, H., Llorens-Cortes, C., and Schwartz, J. Enkephalin receptors on dopaminergic neurones in rat striatum. *Nature* 268, 745-747 (1977).
102. Pomeranz, B., Cheng, R., and Law, P. Acupuncture reduces electrophysiological and behavioral responses to noxious stimuli: Pituitary is implicated. *Exp. Neurol.* 54, 172-178 (1977).
103. Pomeranz, B. and Chiu, D. Naloxone blockade of acupuncture analgesia: Endorphin implicated. *Life Sci.* 19, 1757-1762 (1976).
104. Puig, M., Gascon, P., Craviso, G., and Musacchio, J. Endogenous opiate receptor ligand: Electrically induced release in the guinea pig ileum. *Science* 195, 419-420 (1977).
105. Queen, G., Pinsky, C., and LaBella, F. Subcellular localization of endorphin activity in bovine pituitary and brain. *Biochem. Biophys. Res. Commun.* 72, 1021-1027 (1976).
106. Ree, J., de Wied, D., Bradbury, A., Hulme, E., Smyth, D., and Snell, C. Induction of tolerance to the analgesic action of lipotropin C-fragment. *Nature* 264, 792-793 (1976).
107. Reynolds, D. Surgery in the rat during electrical analgesia induced by focal brain stimulation.

Science 164, 444-445 (1969).

108. Roemer, D., Buescher, H., Hill, R., Pless, J., Bauer, W., Cardinaux, F., Closse, A., Hauser, D., and Huquenin, R. A synthetic enkephalin analogue with prolonged parenteral and oral analgesic activity. *Nature* 268, 547-549 (1977).

109. Ronai, A., Szekely, J., Graf, L., Dunai-Kovacs, Z., and Bajusz, S. Morphine-like analgesic effect of a pituitary hormone, β-lipotropin. *Life Sci.* 19, 733-378 (1976).

110. Rossier, J., French, E.D., Rivier, C., Ling, N., Guillemin, R., and Bloom, F.E. Foot-shock induced stress increases β-endorphin levels in blood but not brain. *Nature* 270, 618-620 (1977).

111. Schmidt, R.F. Control of the access of afferent activity to somatosensory pathways, in *Handbook of Sensory Physiology. VII. Somatosensory System.* A. Iggo, ed. Springer, Berlin, 1973, pp. 151-206.

112. Segal, D., Browne, R., Bloom, F., Ling, N., and Guillemin, R. β-endorphin: endogenous opiate or neuroleptic? *Science* 198, 411-414 (1977).

113. Seidah, N., Dragon, N., Benjannet, S., Routhier, R., and Chretien, M. The complete sequence of sheep beta-endorphin. *Biochem. Biophys. Res. Commun.* 74, 1528-1535 (1977).

114. Simantov, R., and Snyder, S. Isolation and structure identification of a morphine-like peptide "enkephalin" in bovine brain. *Life Sci.* 18, 781-788 (1976).

115. Simon, E.J., Hiller, J.M., and Edelman, I. Stereospecific binding of the potent narcotic analgesic 3H-etorphine to rat brain homogenate. *Proc. Nat. Acad. Sci. USA* 70, 1947-1949 (1973).

116. Simon, E., Hiller, J., Groth, J., and Edelman, I. Further properties of stereospecific opiate binding sites in rat brain: On the nature of the sodium effect. *Pharmacol. Exp. Ther.* 192, 531-537 (1976).

117. Smith, T.W., Hughes, J., Kosterlitz, H.W., and Sosa, R.P. Enkephalins: Isolation, distribution and function, in *Opiates and Endogenous Opioid Peptides.* H.W. Kosterlitz, ed. North Holland, Amsterdam, 1976, pp. 57-62.

118. Snyder, S. Opiate receptor in normal and drug altered brain function. *Nature* 257, 185-189 (1975).

119. Snyder, S. Discussion, in, S. Reichlin, R.J. Baldessarini, and J.B. Martin, eds. *The Hypothalamus.* Raven Press, New York, 1978, p. 248.

120. Szekely, J., Ronai, A., Dunai-Kovacs, Z., Miglecz, E., Bajusz, S., and Graf, L. Cross tolerance between morphine and β-endorphin in vivo. *Life Sci.* 20, 1259-1264 (1977).

121. Terenius, L. Stereospecific interaction between narcotic analgesics and a synaptic plasma membrane fraction of rat cerebral cortex. *Acta Pharmacol. Toxicol.* 32, 317-320 (1973).

122. Terenius, L. and Wahlstrom, A. A morphine-like ligand for opiate receptors in human CSF. *Life Sci.* 16, 1759-1764 (1975).

123. Terenius, L. and Wahlstrom, A. Search for an endogenous ligand for the opiate receptor. *Acta Physiol. Scand.* 94, 74-81 (1975).

124. Terenius, L., Wahlstrom, A., Lindstrom, L., and Widerlov, E. Increased CSF levels of endorphins in chronic psychosis. *Neurosci. Lett.* 3, 157-162 (1976).

125. Teschemacher, H., Opheim, K., Cox, B., and Goldstein, A. A peptide-like substance from pituitary that acts like morphine. *Life Sci.* 16, 1771-1776 (1975).

126. Tseng, L-F., Loh, H., and Li, C. β-endorphin as a potent analgesic by intravenous injection. *Nature* 263, 239-240 (1976).

127. Tseng, L-F., Loh, H., and Li, C. Human β-endorphin: Development of tolerance and behavioral activity in rats. *Biochem. Biophys. Res. Commun.* 74, 390-396 (1977).

128. Urca, G., Frenk, H., Liebeskind, J., and Taylor, A. Morphine and enkephalin: Analgesic and epileptic properties. *Science* 197, 83-86 (1977).

129. Veith, J.L., Sandman, C.A., Walker, J.M., Coy, D.H., and Kastin, A.J. Endorphins:

Systematic administration selectively alters open field behavior of rats. *Pharmacol. Biochem. Behav.* 20, 539-542 (1978).

130. Volavka, J., Mallya, A., Baig, S., Perez-Cruet, J. Naloxone in chronic schizophrenia. *Science* 196, 1227-1228 (1977).

131. Walker, J., Berntson, G., Sandman, C., Coy, D., Schally, A., and Kastin, A. An analog of enkephalin having prolonged opiate-like effects in vivo. *Science* 196, 85-87 (1977).

132. Walker, J.M., Sandman, C.A., Berntson, C.G., McGivern, R.F., Coy, D.H., and Kastin, A.J. Endorphin analogs with potent and long-lasting analgesic effects. *Pharmacol. Biochem. Behav.* 7, 543-548 (1977).

133. Waterfield, A., Hughes, J., and Kosterlitz, H. Cross tolerance between morphine and methionine-enkephalin. *Nature* 260, 624-625 (1976).

134. Wei, E. and Loh, H. Physical dependence on opiate-like peptides. *Science* 193, 1262-1263 (1976).

135. Zieglgansberger, W., Fry, J.P., Moroder, L., Hertz, A., and Wunsch, E. Enkephalin-induced inhibition of cortical neurones and the lack of this effect in morphine tolerant/dependent rats. *Brain Res.* 115, 160-164 (1976).

CHAPTER 3

Radiological Imaging of Causes of Spinal Pain

BERT LINCOLN PEAR

INTRODUCTION

The spinal cord is encased in an articulated protective cloak of bone. Pain fibers from the posterior spinal roots ascend in the lateral spinothalamic tracts, but the cord—like the brain—is insensitive to pain. Instead, pain is perceived as a sensation arising from mechanoreceptors related to the spinal dura, the periosteum of the surrounding bone, the spinal ligaments, the outer layers of the annulus fibrosus of the discs, and to the venous plexuses and arteries within the epidural space. Stimuli from the overlying skin, surrounding muscles and fascia, and from the spinal apophyseal joints are transmitted through the posterior ramus of the segmental nerve and by the sinuvertebral nerve—the nerve of Luschka. Mechanical deformation of the nerve roots within the subarachnoid and subdural spaces and intervertebral foramen also causes pain.

The sensation of pain is subjective, but pain evokes objective signs and is provoked by recognizable pathological processes. Many of these are demonstrable by the varied modalities of radiological imaging. The initial radiological examination for detection of the source of spinal pain is invariably the conventional roentgenogram. This delineates the vertebral bodies, the vertebral articulations, and the sacroiliac joints. In this way many of the congenital, metabolic, traumatic, inflammatory, neoplastic and degenerative afflictions of the spine can be detected.

CONGENITAL ANOMALIES

A major group of anomalies relates to altered segmentation in keeping with a phylogenetic reduction in the number of vertebrae from lower mammals to man. This group includes assimilation of the atlas to the occiput, fused vertebrae, sacralization of L5, and lumbarization of S1.

In a second group the malformation occurs in the longitudinal plane and there is a failure of fusion in the midline resulting in dysraphism or rachischisis. Spina bifida occulta and neural arch defects are examples.

A less common third category occurs when there is failure of fusion of the two primitive sclerotomes which form the vertebral body, resulting in a coronal cleft body.

A great deal of temerity is required in attempting to evaluate the relationship of minor congenital variations to low back and sciatic pain. Anomalies are common and their significance is in doubt.

George found congenital anomalies in 35% of spines (9). Willis noted that numerical variations are frequent and 10% of humans have a tendency toward unilateral or bilateral sacralization of the last lumbar vertebrae, another 10% have lumbarization of the first sacral segment, while 6 to 7% have a defective neural arch. This, he points out, is strikingly similar to the incidence of 27% of lumbosacral anomalies found by Hodges and Peck in a group of 447 patients with low back pain and sciatic nerve radiation (12).

At the end of World War II, Southworth and Bersack studied anomalies of the lumbosacral vertebrae in 550 veterans who had no symptoms referable to the lower back. Of these 26.5% had asymmetry of the articular facets at L-4, 17.4% at L-5, S-1, 18.2% had spina bifida occulta, 6.4% sacralization of the last lumbar vertebra, 2% lumbarization of the first sacral segment, 11% had lumbar ribs, and 22% had scoliosis (28).

Evaluation of available data suggests that pain may be related to disc degeneration or apophyseal joint arthritis in those abnormalities where there is abnormal motion of one vertebra upon another. These include hemivertebra, fused vertebra, hypoplasia or aplasia of an articular facet and spondylolisthesis.

SPONDYLOLISTHESIS

Spondylolysis is a defect in the neural arch of a lumbar vertebra, generally L-5. This allows varying degrees of forward subluxation of one segment upon the other, termed spondylolisthesis* (slipped vertebra). The dislocation can be minimal or extreme and L-5 can come to rest in front of S-1.

There is a paradox in the assertion that spondylolisthesis is the most frequent symptomatic congenital abnormality, since there is no unanimity as to its cause (5). Acquired spondylolisthesis has followed spinal fusion, stress infraction, and acute trauma. It may appear in repetitive extension injuries such as occur in professional football linemen.

Nonetheless, spondylolisthesis also appears to have a genetic background and is often associated with anomalies such as spina bifida, gracile neural arches or elongated pars interarticulares. There may be both a congenital and a traumatic causation (5).

The affected vertebral body frequently has a trapezoid configuration with a diminished posterior height. The defect in the pars interarticularis is usually seen on the routine films, but oblique tomograms are occasionally necessary for definitive delineation. Myelography distinguishes those cases in which symptoms are related to vertebral encroachment upon the dural sac and nerve roots from those which are related to disc herniation.

ARTHRITIDES

Of the many arthritides, ankylosing spondylitis most frequently involves the spine and sacroiliac joints. Its onset is generally in the second or third decade of life with a predominantly male incidence. The association of the disease with high titers of HLA-W27 antigen is now well established.

Ankylosing spondylitis often presents with episodes of low back pain and aching in the sacroiliac and hip joints. Sciatic radiation occurs in a significant number of patients and disc disease is initially suspected until radiographic evidence of joint disease is found on routine films or at myelography.

The arthritis first involves the iliac side of the sacroiliac joints. There is patchy osteoporosis with loss of the integrity of the normal thin white cortical margin of the subchondral bone. Subsequently there is blurring and fraying of the cortical margins of the joint followed by focal areas of sclerosis eventuating in bony joint fusion. The sequence is that of inflammation, reaction, and then repair.

---

*Degenerative spondylolisthesis with an intact neural arch has a different genesis and represents vertebral subluxation due to degenerative arthritis of the apophyseal joints with or without disc degeneration.

In the spine the apophyseal joints and costovertebral joints are involved in an ascending direction. The earliest changes in the vertebral bodies are erosions of the anterior corners, resulting in "squaring" of the vertebral contour. As the disease progresses, there is ossification of adjacent bodies, predominantly in the outer layers of the annulus fibrosus and contiguous bone. Laterally there is formation of bony bridges known as syndesmophytes.

A form of ankylosing spondylitis occurs in association with intestinal inflammatory disease and is identical with the idiopathic type. This association with ulcerative colitis and Crohn's disease is more common than would be expected solely by chance. The sacroiliitis and spondylitis usually develop after the intestinal disease, but may precede it or have a synchronous onset.

Sacroiliitis also occurs with psoriasis and in Reiter's disease. Involvement may be bilateral and symmetrical, bilateral but asymmetrical, or unilateral, as contrasted to ankylosing spondylitis where it is symmetrical. In the spine the syndesmophytes are usually asymmetrical and nonmarginal. The pattern of these diseases in other joints differs from each other and also from ankylosing spondylitis.

Other arthritides also involve the sacroiliac joints and cause low back pain. These are as variegated as degenerative arthritis, rheumatoid arthritis, gout, infection, ochronosis, relapsing polychondritis, Familial Mediterranean Fever, and lipoid dermatoarthritis.

NUCLEAR IMAGING

Prominent uptake of radioactive technetium-99m bone-seeking polyphosphate compounds is normal within the sacroiliac joints. This increases in sacroiliitis and may precede recognizable roentgen signs.

Conversely, increased uptake does not occur in osteitis condensans ilii where there is a variable degree of dense sclerosis on the iliac side of the joint. Osteitis is a misnomer, since it is not an inflammation but a stress eburnation generally found in multiparous young women.

METASTATIC NEOPLASM

Metastatic neoplastic disease is a major cause of back pain and this symptom cannot be ignored in a patient with a known primary tumor. There is a predilection for red marrow and within bone the spine is the most common site for metastases. A major route of spread is by the vertebral venous plexus of Batson. This sluggish, valveless venous system extends along the spine from the pelvis to the dural sinuses and communicates with the jugular, brachiocephalic, axillary, intercostal, azygous, and other veins.

Batson's veins must play a role in the deposition of tumor cells from cancer of the breast, prostate, and lung to the spine. These neoplasms and those arising from the kidney, thyroid, and bowel are the primary source for over three-fourths of bony metastases. The eventual incidence of osseous spread from all cancers has been variably estimated as between 27 to 40% (1). Higher occurrences are found in carcinoma of the breast in women and carcinoma of the prostate in men. For lung cancer the incidence has been said to range from 15 to 44% (18). Osseous metastases are detected in about 15% of the cases of Hodgkin's disease during life and a higher percentage is found at postmortem examination (25). Sarcomas, including those arising in bone, also metastasize to the skeleton.

One of the earliest recognizable roentgen signs of spinal involvement is destruction of a vertebral pedicle. This finding is so consistent that meticulous attention must be directed to evaluation of the integrity of the pedicles in any spinal examination. The majority of metastatic lesions are smaller than primary bone tumors when first discovered, are multiple, have no tumor matrix, and evoke periosteal reaction less often.

FORMS OF BONE DESTRUCTION

Lytic bone lesions are the most common. The form of dissolution depends upon the aggressiveness of the tumor and the host response. Lodwick describes three types of destruction (14-16). Permeative destruction correlates with dissemination and is characterized by tiny holes without clearly definable edges. It is often indistinguishable from an exaggerated trabecular pattern. Moth-eaten destruction is of intermediate aggressiveness with multiple holes of moderate size which tend to coalesce. The zone of transition from abnormal to normal is relatively broad. Geographic destruction suggests a slower process and the hole in bone is relatively large and well defined. The zone of transition is sharp and may even be sclerotized or expansile.

Tumor does not destroy bone in the sense that a mouse eats cheese. Rather it stimulates an osteoclastic response within the bone. However, in other tumors, the presence of neoplastic cells within the bone instead evokes an osteoblastic or osteosclerotic reaction, with formation of new bone upon the surface of preexisting trabeculae diminishing the marrow spaces and creating the radiographic appearance of sclerosis. This occurs in most cases of carcinoma of the prostate and in many breast tumors, but also in virtually any other neoplasm, especially carcinoid, urinary bladder, mucinous cell carcinomas, Hodgkin's disease and medulloblastoma. Why some tumors are lytic and others osteoblastic is not known.

There is a latent period in which bone destruction is undetectable radiographically. Lodwick has shown that significant amounts of cancellous bone can be removed without detection if the cortex is not penetrated. This is particularly true in osteoporotic bone where the trabecular pattern is already sparse (14). Consequently, when there is unexplained pain with suspicion of bony metastases, nuclear scanning is a much more sensitive modality than radiology. It should also be used prior to extensive surgery, even without pain, for those tumors which have a propensity to extend to bone.

NUCLEAR BONE SCANNING

Present day third generation bone scanning utilizes Technetium-99m labeled polyphosphates (*Tc-Polyphosphate, *Tc-Pyrophosphate and *Tc-Diphosphonate). Short-term uptake of these bone seeking radionuclides is closely correlated with blood flow and ion exchange at highly vascularized bone surfaces (8). It is overly simplistic to suggest that increased nuclide uptake is merely related to increased osteoblastic activity, but this is a useful pragmatic clinical theorem.

Brucer conjectures that a 5 to 10% increase in osteogenesis can be detectable on a bone scan. He estimates that in malignant metastatic disease the radiogram and scan agree in about 80% of cases, the x-ray is falsely negative in 16%, while the scan is falsely negative in 4% (2). False negative scans with positive radiograms are generally due to highly anaplastic tumors, some plasma cells myelomas, and occasional indolent tumors which invade the skeleton without reactive bone formation.

Positive nuclear scans also occur in a large variety of benign conditions, including fractures, osteomyelitis, arthritis, Paget's disease, and osteoid osteoma, among many others. Correlative x-rays are therefore essential when a bone scan is positive.

PRIMARY TUMORS OF THE VERTEBRAE

Pain is the principal symptom of primary neoplasms originating in the vertebral column. The single most common solitary tumor of the spine is not a primary one but a metastatic carcinoma. This may appear before the primary source becomes evident.

Virtually any tumor of bone can arise within the spine. This includes chondrosarcoma, osteochondroma, Ewing's sarcoma, osteogenic sarcoma, and hemangioma. Of tumors originating in bone, only chordoma is limited to the spine. This is a locally invasive tumor which arises from notochordal remnants and is most frequently found in the sacrum, then in the clivus, and more rarely in the cervical spine and other vertebrae. Up to 10% may metastasize.

There are three lesions which are not limited to the spine but have a unique localization within the vertebral processes. These are osteoid osteoma, osteoblastoma, and aneurysmal bone cyst. All are benign and usually appear within the first three decades of life.

The nidus of osteoid osteoma is a small round or oval radiolucency frequently surrounded by varying amounts of dense reactive sclerosis and may only be demonstrated by tomography. The pain of this lesion is often dramatically relieved by aspirin.

About half of the cases of osteoblastoma arise within the vertebral column and are related to the neural arch. The tumor is radiolucent and expansile. It tends to be well circumscribed and frequently contains calcium within its stroma.

Aneurysmal bone cyst may be a true tumor or a reaction to injury. Occasionally it may mask an underlying more significant lesion. It can arise within the vertebral body and lead to collapse or originate within a lamina or transverse or spinous process. The lesion results in expansile rarefaction of bone with a fine delimiting shell of cortex which may be so thin as to only be visualized by tomography. Unlike osteoblastoma, there is no calcification within the matrix.

MULTIPLE MYELOMA

Tumors arising within the hematopoietic marrow, such as myelogenous leukemia and reticulum cell sarcoma of bone, are classified as primary bone tumors. Multiple myeloma is therefore characterized as a bone tumor although extraosseous sites are rarely involved.

The spine is more often affected by myeloma than any other part of the skeleton. Pain in the thorax and back is at first vague and generalized. It increases with progressive destruction of bone and with vertebral fracture and nerve root compression.

The disease can initially appear to be "solitary," but dissemination is the rule. The usual findings are widespread osteolytic lesions with little host reaction—the moth-eaten pattern. Destruction of a vertebral body with sparing of the pedicles occurs with statistical relevance more often than in metastatic carcinoma (13). Involvement of long and small bones of the extremities is also more common. Soft tissue masses about destroyed vertebrae and ribs are more prominent than in carcinoma.

Multiple myeloma is rarely osteoblastic. When this occurs, the diagnosis of metastatic carcinoma is usually first entertained.

Generalized osteoporosis can be the only roentgen finding and is related to earlier diagnosis. Since myeloma and osteoporosis are found in the same general age group, this sign is difficult to interpret. The problem can be readily resolved by gamma globulin electrophoresis. If a M spike is found, bone marrow studies can then be obtain (20).

SPINAL CORD TUMORS

Intraspinal neoplasms comprise a group quite distinct from those arising from the bony spine. The presence of pain as a prominent symptom varies with the site of origin of the tumor. It predominates in neurofibromas which arise from nerve roots and in intramedullary ependymomas of the filum terminale which encroach upon the cauda equina. About 4 to 5.6% of patients suspected of having a protruded intervertebral disc are found to have a tumor of the spinal cord at operation (4, 17).

Intramedullary tumors arise from the cord substance and represent between 10 to 20% of neural column tumors. Most are gliomas, either ependymomas or astrocytomas, but rarely glioblastomas.

The slowly growing tumors, particularly in the young, produce plain film changes with widening of the spinal canal, posterior scalloping of the vertebral bodies and pressure erosion of the pedicles. The diagnosis is invariably established by myelography. There is fusiform expansion of the spinal cord, greatest at the center of the tumor. This narrows the spinal subarachnoid space and eventually occludes it.

Syringomyelia produces similar fusiform expansion of the spinal cord. Distinction is possible at air myelography. Gravitational changes occur in the shape of the cystic syrinx but not in solid neoplasms with changes in position of the patient.

Arteriovenous malformations occur within the cord and also produce a mass effect. The tortuous plexus of arteries and veins associated with the mass are usually demonstrable at myelography as streaks within the Pantopaque column. The diagnosis is confirmed by spinal angiography, which delineates the origin and extent of the feeding and draining vessels.

Distinction must be made between arteriovenous malformation and hemangioblastoma which is a true tumor of the spinal cord. The latter is usually associated with greater mass while the vessels conform to a smaller nidus.

INTRADURAL-EXTRAMEDULLARY TUMORS

Intradural-extramedullary tumors constitute more than half of neural canal neoplasms and are almost equally divided between neurofibromas and meningiomas. Less commonly congenital and acquired epidermoid inclusion cysts occur in this location (21, 22). These tumors are of particular importance since they are benign and there is excellent potential for complete cure.

Neurofibromas arise from the nerve sheath in any portion of the spinal cord. They generally occur in younger patients with an equal ratio in both sexes. Many of the tumors pass through an intervertebral foramen into the paraspinous space, causing enlargement of the canal. This and other bony changes are four times more common with neurofibroma than with meningioma.

The spinal tumors are often multiple when associated with generalized neurofibromatosis. Characteristic defects in the bony orbit, congenital bowing and pseudoarthrosis, severe scoliosis, and intrathoracic meningoceles are present in a large percentage of patients with Von Recklinghausen's disease.

Meningiomas occur most frequently within the dorsal spine of middle aged women. Bony changes are less common than in neurofibroma but calcifications occur in up to one-third of the cases and are virtually diagnostic of meningioma when identified (24).

At myelography the Pantopaque within the subarachnoid space engulfs intradural-extramedullary tumors, producing a sharply defined rounded or lobulated defect representing the mass. The spinal cord is displaced to the opposite side leaving a large free subarachnoid space filled with contrast above the tumor. The floor of this space is formed by the upper margin of the tumor and the Pantopaque rests upon it like a cap. Even if complete obstruction has occurred, the margin of the tumor projecting against the Pantopaque will be outlined as a crescentric or concave defect displacing the spinal cord.

EXTRADURAL TUMORS

Most extradural tumors are malignant implants from carcinoma, lymphoma, or myeloma. In many, bony destructive changes are already evident. Less commonly, teratomas, chordomas, hemangiomas, and even neurofibromas and meningiomas occur in this space.

Sudden pain and neurological deficit can also be produced by bleeding into the spinal epidural space in patients on anticoagulant therapy or with bleeding dyscrasias. Epidural hematoma can also be posttraumatic or postsurgical and on occasion the bleeding may appear to be "spontaneous" (23).

INFECTIVE SPONDYLITIS

A wide variety of processes cause destruction of a vertebral body. When this is associated with disc destruction, the lesion is almost invariably inflammatory. An important, but rare, exception is Hodgkin's disease which can destroy bone and its adjacent disc.

The polymorphonuclear leukocytes associated with pyogenic infections elaborate a chondrolysin which rapidly destroys the cartilage of the disc. In tuberculosis, where the response is monocytic, the disc is more slowly attacked. In both pyogenic and tuberculous spondylitis there are contiguous paraspinous abscesses.

INTERVERTEBRAL DISC DISEASE

Burton, of the Sister Kenny Institute of Minneapolis, quotes statistics indicating that over 7 million persons seek medical attention for low back pain each year. He further states that in 1974, the 2614 neurosurgeons in the United States performed over 117,000 back operations for ruptured discs while the number done by the over 10,000 orthopedic suregeons is not known (3).

The intervertebral disc is a complex structure composed of the hyaline cartilage plate of two adjacent vertebral bodies, a central nucleus pulposus, and an encircling ring of fibrocartilage, the annulus fibrosus. Peripheral fibers of the annulus bind it to the bony rim of the vertebral bodies. Anterior and posterior longitudinal ligaments extend along the ventral and dorsal surface of the vertebral column and lend further support.

The nucleus pulposus can be directly radiogramed after injection of aqueous contrast through the annulus by needle puncture. This procedure is of diminishing utility, but the technic has offered insight into the structure of the disc and its progressive degeneration with disease and senesence.

Disc degeneration results in annular bulging or collapse as the disc space narrows. The process may go no farther. At this point, if discogenic symptoms are present they probably arise from secondary degenerative arthritis due to malalignment of the apophyseal joints or from narrowing of intervertebral foramina due to apposition of the adjacent vertebra.

Disc protrusion or herniation are synonomous and represent another stage. The protrusion can occur into the neighboring vertebra through the cartilaginous plate, producing a Schmorl's node, anteriorly, beneath the anterior longitudinal ligament, or laterally. These protrusions are asymptomatic, but the latter two are probably responsible for osteophytic spurring due to metaplastic new bone at the site of insertion of Sharpey's fibers of the annulus upon the vertebral margins. The nonjudgmental term "osteophyte" seems more appropriate than "spondylosis" for this phenomenon which does not correlate with sciatic pain.

Of greater significance are those protrusions which herniate postero-laterally or posteriorly where the annulus and posterior longitudinal ligaments are weaker. These can cause sciatica and neurological symptoms with or without back pain.

There is a great variability in the size and shape of protrusions into or through the disrupted annulus. The protrusion can be a localized bulge or mound beneath the posterior ligament or a polypoid or pedunculated mass which projects posteriolaterally, directly posteriorly, or which extends into an intervertebral foramen.

Massive extrusions are less common. These either dissect beneath the posterior longitudinal ligament and migrate distally or rupture through the ligament to lie free within the subdural space. Massive extrusion can simulate spinal cord tumor clinically and at myelography.

Protrusions occur at the L5-S1 space slightly more often than at L4-L5, and rarely at L3-L4 and L2-L3. Lesions occur at two levels in about 11% of the cases and are occasionally bilateral at the same level.

Acute cervical discs are most common at C5-C6 and C6-C7. In the cervical spine the pain and radiculopathy may be due to soft extruded disc material or to osteophytic encroachment upon the nerve roots.

CONVENTIONAL RADIOGRAMS

Acute disc herniation can occur without demonstrable plain film findings and without narrowing of the disc space. There may be early dynamic change with inhibition to the normal motility between two vertebrae. Later there is a decrease in the height of the disc, frequently associated with degenerative changes in the apophyseal joints, malalignment, osteophytic lipping, and vacuum disc.

Discogenic vertebral sclerosis with irregularity of the vertebral endplates and narrowing of the disc space can simulate infection. Characteristically, the sclerosis is rounded or hemispheric and located anteriorly within the vertebral body contiguous to the narrowed disc. There is frequently a central lucency within the area of sclerosis and when a vacuum phenomenon occurs this excludes the presence of pus within the disc space (19, 26).

It is difficult to ascertain how frequently surgery is now being performed for protruded intervertebral disc on the basis of clinical signs and symptoms alone. At present most authorities advise myelography prior to disc surgery to verify the exact level, recognize multiple disc herniations, and exclude primary tumors of the conus medullaris and cauda equina as well as metastatic neoplasm.

MYELOGRAPHY

Until recently, myelography in the United States was performed using Pantopaque (iophendylate, Lafayette Pharmaceutical). Now metrizamide, a new nonionic water soluble contrast medium has been approved for use by the Food and Drug Administration and is gaining rapid acceptance in this country.

The Pantopaque is injected into the spinal subarachnoid space by needle puncture and subsequently removed at the conclusion of the examination.

Protruded discs most commonly cause a unilateral indentation upon the anterolateral margin of the subarachnoid Pantopaque which is seen best on oblique views. The size of the indentation varies with the size of the protrusion. Larger protrusions elevate and then obliterate the axillary pouch (also called root pocket) of the corresponding nerve. Often the affected nerve is edematous if it is seen through the Pantopaque column (27).

Central discs crowd the roots of the cauda equina laterally and leave the Pantopaque in a shallow central trough, creating an hour-glass deformity. Massive extrusions occlude the canal and there is a striated or "horse-hair" compression of the theca by the epidural mass.

False negative examinations are due to obscuration of small herniations by the density of the Pantopaque, but even large protrusions are missed when they lie lateral to the opacified subarachnoid column.

Unlike Pantopaque, the new water soluble contrast materials need not be removed following the examination and are absorbed from the cerebrospinal fluid into the blood stream. They are not completely without complication, but a major advantage is that they are less opaque and provide more detailed information of the axillary pouches and the course of the nerve roots within the cul-de-sac. Small herniations produce short discrete compression of the axillary pouch of the nerve root with slight swelling of the affected nerve proximal to the defect; with larger protrusions the pouch is occluded and the nerve swollen for a distance of 1 to 2 cm.

EPIDURAL VENOGRAPHY

The vertebral veins consist of an external and internal venous plexus. The latter surrounds the dura along the course of the spine. Intervertebral veins connect the two plexuses. When disc protrusion is suspected and the clinical and myelographic findings are equivocal or the latter normal, additional information may be obtained by epidural venography best performed by venous catheter technique. Disc herniation causes compression or obstruction of the internal epidural vein at the affected level.

FAILURE OF DISC SURGERY

Disc surgery for sciatic pain is not uniformly successful. Failures are relatively common with residual back pain, nerve root symptoms, or functional impairment in as many as 37.7% of the patients evaluated ten or more years after simple disc escision (6, 7). The success of the surgery largely depends upon whether an offending prolapse is found and removed. This in turn relates to preoperative accuracy of diagnosis. When Hirsch and Nachemson analyzed their patients with sciatica, disc prolapse was found in 89% when there were also positive neurological signs and a positive Lasèque leg raising test. The accuracy increased to 90% if the preoperative myelogram was also positive. When prolapse was present the percentage of those not improved by surgery was only 4%, while this was 30% when herniation was not present (11). It must be emphasized that many of their patients who were "improved" still had residual symptoms of varying degree and intensity.

In that same study, 90% of the patients with a positive myelogram had confirmed disc prolapse at surgery. In 8% the myelographic abnormality was due to adhesions, scar, or fibrosis around a nerve root. In the remaining 2% no cause could be found to explain the radiographic abnormality.

However when there was the clinical triad of sciatica, appropriate neurological findings, and a postive Lasèque sign, there was still a 55% probability of disc herniation even with a negative myelogram.

THE FAILED BACK SURGERY SYNDROME (FBSS)

There are many causes for surgical failure in disc disease, i.e., FBSS. The common causes of failure after disc excision with fusion is pseudoarthrosis of the graft or spinal stenosis secondary to graft hypertrophy. In patients with simple disc escision only, recurrent disc extrusion or soft tissue scarring are often responsible.

Failures result if the initial diagnosis was in error. Many patients are characterized as having a "ruptured disc" when in actuality the symptoms are due to other causes of nerve root compression. Encroachment with constriction occur not only within the intervertebral foramen but also at its point of exit secondary to thinning of the disc and approximation of the pedicles. Anterior bony spur formation from adjacent vertebrae and posterior hypertrophic degenerative arthritis of the apophyseal joints also compress spinal nerves and the sinuvertebral nerve of Luschka. These formerly occult stenoses are now demonstrable by CT scanning, particularly when sagittal reconstruction of the image can be obtained.

SPINAL STENOSIS

Stenosis of the spinal canal and foramen can be congenital or acquired, localized or diffuse. Acquired localized stenosis of the cervical spine is generally related to central disc bulging and osteophyte, producing a compressive transverse bar upon the spinal cord. This is frequently associated with narrowing of the intervertebral foramen by osteophytes or disc protrusions and often by hypertrophy of the ligamenta flava. Radiographically narrowing of the antero-posterior diameter of the canal to 13 mm is significant, although myelopathy and radicular pain can occur with larger dimensions.

Diffuse congenital narrowing of the lumbar spine can cause episodes of low back pain with development of spinal claudication, particularly as aging and disc degeneration results in further constriction by annular bulging and hypertrophic spurring. Congenital stenosis is recognizable not only by narrowing of the dimensions of the spinal canal, but the pedicles of the vertebrae are short and thick and the laminae and facet joints have a characteristic vertical inclination, often tilted inward and overlapping. This differs from the X shape of divergent normal laminae and apophyseal joints. Myelography demonstrates a constricted canal with crowding of the nerve roots within the subarachnoid space, compression, and even obstruction.

ARACHNOIDITIS

Lumbosacral arachnoiditis must be included in the gamut of causes of constant and often incapacitating low back and leg pain following disc surgery.

Arachnoiditis is an inflammatory reaction of the pia-arachnoid. It was classically described as the result of pyogenic, tuberculous, or luetic infection. At present, most cases appear to be due to the irritative effects of trauma, disc prolapse, surgery, and intrathecal blood and foreign substances in varied combination. Spinal anesthesia, Pantopaque, and water-soluble contrast media have all be indicted.

Burton in 1978, studied 100 patients with adhesive arachnoiditis documented either by surgery or by myelography. The group averaged 2.8 Pantopaque examinations and 3.6 back operations per patient, indicating that this is one of the major causes of the FBSS (3).

Characterization of arachnoiditis by Pantopaque myelography includes an appearance of "candle guttering" with irregular pockets of contrast, deformation of the normal striations of cauda equina and often obstruction. The diagnosis is not unequivocal and extra-arachnoid injection, spinal stenosis, and dural and perineural scar can be misinterpreted as arachnoiditis.

The inflammation results in agglutination of the nerve roots and their axillary pouches (root pockets). This is more exquisitely delineated by the less dense and less viscid water-soluble contrast media than with Pantopaque. The signs are felt to be (1) nonfilling of the axillary pouches, usually symmetrically; (2) disappearance of the normal striation of the cauda equina; and (3) narrowing of the caudal sac (10). These are to be distinguished from incomplete filling of a single axillary pouch at the site of operation as the result of postsurgical scar.

The role of Pantopaque in the causation of arachnoiditis has not yet been resolved. Myelography is an important and necessary diagnostic procedure. Almost half a million Pantopaque myelograms are performed each year and the incidence of arachnoiditis is quite minimal following uncomplicated myelography not followed by surgery. Water-soluble media may reduce this further, but these do have short-term complications of nausea, headache, spasm, hypotension, and seizures.

An increasing role is predicted for noninvasive CT scanning.

CONCLUSION

Radiological imaging is a form of physical diagnosis no different from seeing, listening, or the laying on of hands. The probing photons, gamma rays, and ultrasonic waves are prolongations of the fingers; the x-ray film, fluoroscopic screen and cathode ray tube display are extensions of the retinae. Through these the radiologist perceives normal and morbid anatomy and often function. Although the sensation of pain cannot be visualized, the causes of pain can often be shown.

REFERENCES

1. Abrams, H.L. Skeletal metastases in carcinoma. *Radiology* 55, 534-538 (1950).
2. Brucer, M. A history of bone scanning, in *Vignettes in Nuclear Medicine,* vol. 83. Mallinckrot Inc., St. Louis, 1976, pp. 1-18.
3. Burton, C.V. Lumbosacral arachnoiditis. *Spine* 3, 24-29 (1978).
4. Craig, W.McK., Svien, H.J., Dodge, H.W., Jr., Camp, J.D. Intraspinal lesions masquerading as protruded lumbar intervertebral disks. *J. Am. Med. Assoc.* 149, 250-253 (1952).
5. DePalma, A.F. and Rothman, R.H. *The Intervertebral Disc.* W.B. Saunders, Philadelphia, 1970.
6. Frymoyer, J.W., Hanley, E.N., Howe, J. Kuhlmann, D., Matteri, R. Disc excision and spine fusion in the management of lumbar disc disease: A minimum ten-year follow-up. *Spine* 3, 1-6 (1978).

7. Frymoyer, J.W., Matteri, R.E., Hanley, E.N., Kuhlmann, D., Howe, J. Failed lumbar disc surgery requiring second operation: A long term follow-up study. *Spine* 3, 7-11 (1978).
8. Genant, H.K., Bavtovich, G.J., Singh, M. Bone-seeking radionuclides: In vivo study of skeletal uptake. *Radiology* 113, 373-382 (1974).
9. George, A.W. The vertebrae roentgenologically considered. W.B. Saunders, New York, 1919.
10. Hansen, E.B., Fahrenkrug, A., Praestholm, J. Late meningeal effects of myelographic contrast media with special reference to metrizamide. *Br. J. Radio.* 51, 321-327 (1978).
11. Hirsh, C. and Nachemson, A. The reliability of lumbar disk surgery. *Clin. Orth. P.* 29, 189-194 (1963).
12. Hodges, E.J. and Peck W.S. Clinical and roentgenological study of low back pain with sciatic radiation. *Am. J. Roentgenol.* 37, 461-468 (1937).
13. Jacobson, H.G., Poppel, M.H., Shapiro, J.H., Grossberger, S. The vertebral pedicle sign: A roentgen finding to differentiate metastatic carcinoma from multiple myeloma. *Am. J. Roentgenol.* 80, 817-821 (1958).
14. Lodwick, G.S. Reactive response to local injury in bone. *Radiol. Clinics North Am.* 2, 209-219 (1964).
15. Lodwick, G.S. A Systemic approach of the roentgen diagnosis of bone tumors, in *Tumors of Bone and Soft Tissue—8th Annual Clinical Conference on Cancer, 1963.* Yearbook Publ., Chicago, 1965.
16. Lodwick, G.S. A probability approach to the diagnosis of bone tumors. *Radio. Clinics North Am.* 3, 487-497 (1965).
17. Love, J.G. and Rivers, M.H. Spinal cord tumors simulating protruded intervertebral disks. *J. Am. Med. Assoc.* 179, 878-88 (1962).
18. Napoli, L.D., Hansen, H.H., Muggia, F.M., and Twigg, H.L. The incidence of osseous involvement in lung cancer with special reference to the development of osteoblastic changes. *Radiology* 108, 17-21 (1973).
19. Martel, W., Seeger, J.F., Wicks, J.D., and Washburn, R.L. Traumatic lesions of the discovertebral junction in the lumbar spine. *Am. J. Roentgenol.* 127, 457-464 (1976).
20. Pear, B.L. The plasma cell in radiology. *Am. J. Roentgenol.* 102, 908-915 (1968).
21. Pear, B.L. Iatrogenic intraspinal epidermoid sequestration cysts. *Radiology* 92, 251-254 (1969).
22. Pear, B.L. Epidermoid and dermoid sequestration cysts. *Am. J. Roentgenol.* 110, 159-165 (1970).
23. Pear, B.L. Spinal epidural hematoma. *Am. J. Roentgenol.* 115, 155-164 (1972).
24. Pear, B.L. and Boyd, H.R. Roentgenographically visible calcifications in spinal meningioma. *Am. J. Roentgenol.* 120, 32-45 (1974).
25. Pear, B.L. Skeletal Manifestations of the lymphomas and leukemias. *Semin. Roentgenol.* 9, 229-240 (1974).
26. Sauser, D.D., Goldman, A.B., and Kaye, J.J. Discogenic vertebral sclerosis. *J. Can. Assoc. Radiol.* 29, 44-50 (1977).
27. Shapiro, R. *Myelography,* 3rd ed. Yearbook Medical Publ., Chicago, 1975.
28. Southworth, J.D. and Bersack, S.R. Anomalies of the lumbosacral vertebrae in five hundred and fifty individuals without symptoms referable to the low back. *Am. J. Roentgenol.* 64, 624-634 (1950).

CHAPTER 4

The Nature of Pain

H. MERSKEY

THE NATURE OF PAIN

Pain does not have a simple one to one relationship with tissue damage or body lesions. This is true even if special anatomical and pathological factors are taken into account. The same amount of damage in the same region produces very different complaints of pain according to the mood of the individual, his social and cultural background, the significance to him of the wound, the circumstances in which it occurs, and so on. The evidence on this score has been ably reviewed by many authors, such as Barber (4), Beecher (5), and Sternbach (17). Merskey and Spear (13) and Merskey (12) also surveyed this literature and the literature which showed a close relationship between certain types of psychiatric illness and the occurrence of pain. These topics are also considered by other contributors to this volume.

To summarize the above, it can be said that anxiety and apprehension, plus personal experience, cultural conditioning, and fear of illness all make pain worse. So, at times, does depression. Indeed, psychological processes may produce pain; this is discussed further below. Factors which relieve pain include all types of calming or anxiolytic procedures, such as relaxation, suggestion, hypnosis, minor tranquilizers, and a variety of psychotherapeutic and behavioral techniques. From the information available, it can be concluded that anxiety with moderate arousal causes pain or increases it. Certain other psychological states may, however, reduce or abolish pain. Schizophrenic patients have less pain proportionately than others and states of very high arousal, such as great excitement in battle, also abolish pain.

The extreme case in which severe pain from gross physical lesions is abolished by the power of the mind is unfortunately very rare. But on a more prosaic level we can note that players in competitive sports frequently sustain injuries which cause them no pain until they leave the field or arena, at which point the pain appears and they limp or nurse the tender and bruised part.

These observations lead us to a fundamental problem with regard to pain. It is normally thought to be a consequence of bodily damage, but in fact is often the consequence of emotional disturbance without any contributory physical causes. For example, the majority of psychiatric outpatients have pain without relevant physical illness (10, 15), numerous medical outpatients have pain for emotional reasons (2, 7), and in general practice 22% of 276 patients had pain for psychological reasons (3). Thus, although we think of pain as prima facie a sign of physical disease, it is also a common sign of psychological illness (16).

It may be thought that "pain" in psychological illness is not the same as "pain" in physical illness. Perhaps the patients mean something different. To take such a view would be to deny the experience of the patients who, whatever its cause, regard their pain as being typical of physical disturbance. An analysis of the language used to describe their pain shows that psychiatric patients with pain, and others, use many terms in common and most of those terms reflect the notion of an organic or pathophysiological change in the tissues (7). In the light of observations like these the following definition of pain was made: "An unpleasant experience which we primarily associate with tissue damage or describe in terms of such damage or both" (11, 13).

The purpose of this definition was to characterize pain operationally as a psychological experience. Of course in many instances it has a physical basis, but it is always an unpleasant subjective experience. The use of the word pain by patients reflects their view that it is that sort of experience typically associated with tissue damage. We learn in childhood that knocks and blows cause a certain type of experience which is described as pain. Thereafter, whether the causes of similar experiences are physical or psychological, they are described in the same way, as pain. Doctors find this hard to accept because they are conditioned to thinking of pain in terms of physical mechanisms. That in turn leads them to say, sometimes, that there is no pain when patients still complain of it, but no physical explantion is found. In the management of pain, the first and overriding rule is that the patient's valid experiences are data from which the doctor or the health professional commences his work. Some pains may certainly be thought to be disproportionate to physical causes. They often are. But that then becomes a reason for psychological investigation and not for denial of the pain.

Nothing that has been said so far should be taken to mean that physiological causes are not important with regard to pain. Moreover the neurophysiological state of the patient with pain of organic origin must be different in some ways from that of patients whose pains have a purely psychological basis. There is some evidence of differences in the biochemical states of patients who have lesions causing pain and those who have pain without lesions (9, 18), but the subjective situation is frequently identical. It is true also that some differences in pain descriptions have been found in accordance with the source of pain. Thus pain from physical lesions tends to be more burning in character than pain associated with psychological illness (1). In a series of psychiatric patients, those without lesions more often mentioned throbbing as characteristic of their complaint (6). Differences have further been shown between the pain of dysmenorrhea and that from an unsatisfactory intrauterine device (14). Trigeminal neuralgia is notoriously different from gall bladder colic. Nevertheless the identities between pain of physical origin and pain of psychological origin are greater than the differences in character.

It appears that there is a common pattern of experience in patients who have pain proportionate to their lesions and in patients who do not have a physical mechanism which is sufficient to explain their pain. This is true even where no physical mechanism at all can be found but a psychiatric cause is evident. It follows that "the nature of pain" has to do with that common pattern. I consider that the common pattern or element is that when we talk of pain we speak of experiences and not of physiological mechanisms. The nature of pain is thus described in the definition which was given above. It is an experience. We think of it as being like the experience we undergo when suffering from trauma, but it can occur without trauma or lesion. It is also unpleasant. There are other types of unpleasant experiences, e.g., nausea, vertigo, but their subjective character is obviously different from that of pain and not tied to the idea of bodily damage. The experience of pain although varied and private is also consistent. Like all subjective experiences there is sometimes doubt in marginal cases as to whether we have something which should be called by another term, such as discomfort. There may also be doubt whether it should be regarded as unpleasant but not painful. However if we decide that we have pain the experience complies with the fundamental requirements of being first, unpleasant and second, like bodily damage.

REFERENCES

1. Agnew, D.C. and Merskey, H. Words of chronic pain. *Pain* 2, 73-81 (1976).
2. Bain, S.T. and Spaulding, W.B. The importance of coding presenting symptoms. *Can. Med. Assoc. J.* 97, 953-959 (1967).
3. Baker, J.W. and Merskey, H. Pain in general practice, *J. psychosom. Res.* 10, 383-387 (1967).
4. Barber, T.X. Toward a theory of pain: Relief of chronic pain by pre-frontal leucotomy, opiates, placebos and hypnosis. *Psychol. Bull.* 56, 430-460 (1959).
5. Beecher, H.K. *Measurement of Subjective Responses. Quantitative Effects of Drugs.* Oxford Univ. Press, New York, 1959.
6. Boyd, D.B. and Merskey, H. A Note on the description of pain and its causes. *Pain,* 5, 1-3 (1978).
7. Devine, R. and Merskey, H. The description of pain in psychiatric and general medical patients. *J. Psychosom. Res.* 9, 311-316 (1965).
8. Glynn, C.J. and Lloyd, J.W. Biochemical changes associated with intractable pain. *Br. Med. J.* 1, 280-281 (1978).
9. Lascelles, P.T., Evans, P.R., Merskey, H., and Sabur, M.A. Plasma cortisol in psychiatric and neurological patients with pain. *Brain* 97, 533-538 (1974).
10. Melzack, R. and Torgerson, W.S. On the language of pain. *Anesthesiology* 34, 50-59 (1971).
11. Merskey, H. An investigation of pain in psychological illness. D.M. Thesis, Oxford, 1964.
12. Merskey, H. Psychological aspects of pain. *Postgrad. Med. J.* 44, 297-306 (1968).
13. Merskey, H. and Spear, F.G. *Pain: Psychological and Psychiatric Aspects.* Balliere, Tindall and Cassell, London, 1967.
14. Reading, A.E. and Newton, J.R. A comparison of primary dysmenorrhea and intrauterine-device related pain. *Pain* 3, 265-276 (1977).
15. Spear, F.G. Pain in psychiatric patients. *J. Psychosom. Res.* 11, 187-193 (1968).
16. Stengel, E. Pain and the psychiatrist. *Med. Press* 243, 28-30 (1960).
17. Sternbach, R.A. *Pain: A Psychophysiological Analysis.* Academic Press, New York, 1968.

CHAPTER 5

The Assessment of Pain*

ADA K. JACOX

I always have some pain...it's hard to describe...at times it's sharp and at times it is okay—like you might have with the flu coming on. (patient with rheumatoid arthritis)

It's like severe hunger pangs...when it gets bad, the worst pain, you can just feel the pressure build up and you can feel it go through you. Sometimes it almost sounds like a penny in a rain barrel, a real tight sound as the gurgling noise goes through and that's when the pain lets up a little bit. (patient with cancer)

The patient looked like he was having pain. He was rolling all over the bed and his face was tight. He said that he didn't have any pain though. (student nurse)

The patient complained of pain but we couldn't find any reason for it. We didn't think she needed medication because she shouldn't have had so much pain. Later, x-rays showed metastasis to the bone. (registered nurse)

---

*Presented at the University of Rochester School of Nursing on October 7, 1977, as the Clare Dennison lecture of the year.

The evaluation of patients' pain is difficult for many reasons. The person experiencing the pain has attitudes toward how one should react to and report pain, attitudes shaped by social and cultural forces as well as by personality characteristics. The person making the assessment also has attitudes about how pain should be tolerated or expressed. The ability of one person to interpret accurately what is being felt by another is vastly complicated when the attitudes of the assessor and the person being assessed vary.

If, for example, the nurse or other health professional expects that when a patient is in pain he will verbally say so, but the patient believes he should bear his pain as long as he possibly can without verbally communicating it, the result will be a miscommunication between the two, with the patient needlessly suffering pain. If, on the other hand, the health professional assumes that anyone who is in pain will demonstrate this through nonverbal behavior such as writhing and restlessness, while the patient attempts to control his nonverbal behavior, the result will be another kind of miscommunication. These two examples do not represent the only kinds of miscommunication, but they are common ones in the assessment of pain.

Any attempt to assess the pain of another must begin with the recognition that pain is a subjective phenomenon. The interpretation of a subjective phenomenon such as pain poses many problems, both for the assessor and for the person experiencing it, because of the many factors that influence the perception, response, and report of subjective events.

Sternbach defines pain as "an abstract concept which refers to (1) a personal, private sensation of hurt; (2) a harmful stimulus which signals current or impending tissue damage; (3) a pattern of responses which operate to protect the organism from harm" (10). Although pain has been widely recognized as a sensation, the subjectivity involved in perceiving and responding to a sensation often is overlooked by clinicians. Hilgard, a psychologist who has long been involved in the study of pain, wrote: "I wish to assert flatly that there is no physiological measure of pain which is either as discriminating of fine differences in stimulus conditions, as reliable upon repetition or as lawfully related to changed conditions, as the subject's verbal report" (8).

Recognition of the fact that a verbal report of pain is more reliable than any physiological indicator does not, however, mean that a person's subjective report of pain is the only means of assessment. As Fordyce notes, pain is not simply what a patient says it is, for at least two reasons (5). One reason is that a patients's knowledge and perception will limit his ability to discriminate what is happening in his body. The patient simply may not have sufficient knowledge to be able to interpret and report it even though he may wish to. Second, in pain expression, as in other kinds of expression of human experiences, verbal and nonverbal behavior often differ, and there is no reason for believing that verbal behavior is more valid or believable than nonverbal behavior. "The discrepancy between what people say and what they do is not simply a question of honesty or candor" (5). For various reasons, people may intentionally or unintentionally try to conceal the amount of pain they are feeling, either exaggerating it or deemphasizing it. Many persons who are experiencing chronic pain, for example, have learned to control the expression of their pain. Hackett (6), a psychiatrist, observes that health professional often expect patients to give open and clear evidence of suffering, such as crying, perspiring and writhing.

> This does not take into account the process of adaptation which occurs with pain as well as with other sensations. When pain lasts days and weeks it either produces stress sufficient to exhaust, deplete and eventually destroy the victim or adaptation occurs. Somehow, either through palliation from drugs, or distraction or stoicism and/or a combination of these and more, the individual manages to endure his pain and carry on limited social transactions despite it. He usually can manage to appear untroubled, to be in no pain. However, it would just be as much a mistake to regard such an individual as exemplifying "la belle indifference" as it would to view him as a malingerer. In evaluating chronic pain, a search for evidence that pain exists is fruitless and irrelevant.

The health professional has the difficult job of trying to assess a subjective event being experienced by another person. This is particularly difficult when a person is consciously or unconsciously trying to control the expression of the sensations being experienced or when verbal and nonverbal behaviors are inconsistent. Complicating this further is the problem of the tremendous variation that exists in how people experience pain, including the fact that the same person may react to pain one way at one time and another way at another time. Abrams, a social worker who has had extensive clinical experience in working with patients with cancer, has reported how patients with cancer change their patterns of communication, depending on the stage of cancer in which they are (1). Abrams observed that in the initial stages, most patients are able to talk freely about their diagnoses with physicians and others and the patient may have an air of optimism. In the advancing stage, the patient may become fearful and avoid the diagnosis as it was discussed in the initial stage. They may not respond to opportunities, even when offered by the physician, to ask about their present situation and they become more passive, accepting, and less demanding. In the terminal stage, "silence becomes the common language, especially in the areas of greatest anxiety" (1), such as fear of pain, dying, and death.

In addition to differences in communication during the course of an illness, there are many sociocultural factors that influence who can express pain, who believe they must tolerate it, under what circumstances can pain be discussed, and so forth. Hardy, for example, notes that "pain experienced in certain parts of the body is culturally more acceptable and brings with it greater sympathetic response than pain from other parts. Pain from the genitalia, rectum and anus, or pain resulting from a fall on the buttocks, do not evoke the sympathetic response that pains do from the head, and extremities, chest, or even from the abdomen. Hence, pain of minor intensity from certain regions of the body are complained of more often than others..." (7).

Clearly, what makes pain assessment so difficult is the wide variation in how it is experienced and reported and the varying attitudes that may be held by the person experiencing it and by the person trying to assess it. In the remainder of this chapter, data from several sources will be presented to exemplify and to elaborate upon this problem. One source of data is patients who were experiencing pain; here the focus is upon how they described it and factors that constrained their descriptions. The second source of data is nurses who were attempting to assess patients' pain. The last part of the chapter will include some suggestions regarding how nurses can improve their abilities to evaluate patients' pain.

PAIN FROM THE PATIENT'S POINT OF VIEW

The first set of data is from 102 patients who were experiencing one of three kinds of pain. The first kind of pain is short term, or that experienced by patients undergoing elective surgery such as cholecystectomy and / or herniorrhaphy. The "short term" refers to the pain experienced for the few days or few weeks following surgery. The second group of patients were those experiencing long term pain associated with rheumatoid arthritis. "Long term" refers to pain which patients expect to have for a number of years, but is not necessarily associated with impending death. The third group of patients were those experiencing progressive pain, pain associated with metastatic cancer. For this group of patients, the pain frequently became progressively worse and for many of the patients was associated with impending death. We interviewed these patients regarding how they experienced and reported pain (see ref. 9). One interest was whether and how patients discuss their pain. A question asked was "Do you like to discuss your pain with others?" Table 1 presents the patients' responses. Seventy percent or more of the patients in each group either said no, they did not like to discuss their pain with others or that they were ambivalent about doing so.

A second question asked of those patients who said they do not like to talk with others about their pain was why they did not. Table 2 summarizes these responses.

Table 1. Patients' Preferences with Regard to Discussing Pain*

	Pain group		
Preference	Short term (%) $n=27$	Long term (%) $n=20$	Progressive (%) $n=30$
No	39	45	33
Yes	30	25	27
Uncertain	31	30	40

*Data are from ref. 9.

Table 2. Reasons Why Patients Do Not Talk with Others about their Pain

	Pain group		
Reason	Short term (%) $n=9$	Long term (%) $n=12$	Progressive (%) $n=17$
Does not want sympathy	11.1	16.7	11.8
Others have their own problems or not interested in mine	44.4	41.6	23.5
Social stigma attached to complaining	0	8.3	35.3
Other or did not give a reason	44.4	33.3	29.4

Data are from ref. 9.

The greatest number of patients in both the short term and long term groups said that other people have their own problems and are not interested in learning about someone else's. Responses typical of this category are: "I figure other people have got problems and probably more problems than I've got." "I try to change the subject. Nobody wants to hear about your aches and pains" and "I learned that it isn't the best thing because people aren't interested. When they say 'how are you?' they don't really mean how are you." These were all patients in the short and long term groups. While some of the cancer patients indicated that others were not interested in their pain, some gave responses that are slightly different, in that they suggest that there is a social stigma attached to complaining about pain. More than one-third of the patients in the progressive group gave this negative social labeling as their reason for not discussing their pain with others. Examples of some of these responses are: "I rarely discuss it unless someone asks me. I am not one of those hypochondriacs" and "No one likes a complainer."

In summary, 30% or less of the patients in the three groups said that they like to discuss their pain with others. While some patients described how helpful it was for them to discuss pain with others, many said they preferred not to discuss it or gave somewhat ambivalent or conditional replies, such as "It depends on who is asking me about it." The patients most often gave as reasons for not discussing their pain the belief that people generally are not interested in hearing about someone's pain, and that complaining about pain is negatively valued socially.

Earlier I observed that nurses have difficulty in assessing pain when patients don't show visible signs of it. We asked patients how they usually respond to pain. Nearly two-thirds of the total group reported that they try to remain calm or not to show when they experience pain. The two-thirds include people who make comments such as "I know that its not going to last forever and that it will pass or I will become able to tolerate it, so I kind of wait until it passes." "I ignore it as much as I can" and "I pay as little attention to it as possible." In these and similar responses, patients did not mention feelings of discomfort, anxiety, and so forth, but only commented that they respond to pain by trying to accept or tolerate it.

Other patients specifically mentioned that the pain distresses them but that they try not to show it. Some examples of these responses are: "I usually am pretty tough. I don't like to have anybody see me cry because I'm kind of stubborn." "All you can do is just lie there and suffer it out. There is no sense in putting on a big show or anything like that" and "I try to ignore it until it sort of overcomes me and I couldn't believe there was such severe pain...I guess overall I just retreat and suffer silently."

These responses indicate that most people respond to pain by trying either to ignore it or to conceal it from others. Pain is apparently viewed by many people as a private experience that one tries to keep to oneself. This suggests that, for whatever reasons, many patients will not verbally communicate that they are in pain until the pain is very severe, and some may not verbally communicate it at all.

Probably the most common way in which nurses deal with patients' pain in hospital settings is to assume that when a patient has pain he will say so and then the nurse will check to see whether the PRN medication is due. Clearly, many patients will not communicate that they are in pain and will make strong efforts to conceal it. The process of pain assessment requires active effort on the part of the nurse.

In studying this group of patients it also became apparent that, even when being actively questioned about their pain, patients' understandings of what they were being questioned about differed from what the interviewers thought they were questioning them about. At the beginning of each interview, patients were asked whether or not they were currently in pain. Ten or fifteen minutes later patients were given a sheet of paper with a six-point pain scale, with a zero indicating no pain, 1 mild pain, 2 discomforting, 3 distressing, 4 horrible, and 5 excruciating. Twenty-five percent of the patients who indicated that they were not in pain when asked the direct question later checked on the pain scale either a 1 or a 2, indicating that they were experiencing mild or discomforting pain. For some patients, what they experienced was not identified as pain if it was only mild or discomforting. The question raised by this finding is, if it was not pain, what was it? Subsequent to these descriptive studies of patients' pain, we began a program in which we were testing several interventions to reduce pain. The clinicians working on these projects noted two things: one was that the standardized measures that we were using to measure pain did not always capture the essence of pain, and second, that while some patients may have indicated that the intervention did not reduce their pain, it was producing relief of some kind of distressing symptom.

We then conducted a study to try to determine which experience patients define as painful, which as discomforting, and which as neither. Several pilot studies were done in which approximately 50 patients were asked to describe what they considered to be painful events and what kinds of things were considered to produce discomfort. From their responses, 30 events or conditions were listed and 200 additional patients were asked to classify each condition in terms of whether or not they had ever experienced it and, if they had experienced it, whether they characterized it as pain, discomfort, or neither. In selecting the experiences to include in the final questionnaire, we tried to include some from each of the following categories: those which were primarily physically oriented, such as muscle spasms and those which were more psychosocially oriented such as lack of kindness/consideration on the part of care-takers. We also included conditions and procedures that might be experienced by hospitalized patients, such as insertion of tubes, incisional pain, etc., and experiences that may be common for nonhospitalized persons, such as a headache or slamming a finger in a door. There was no attempt to sample equally from these categories.

The ages of the convenience sample of 200 patients in this study ranged from 16 to 82. Ninety-two were female and 108 male. Forty-five percent were surgical patients and 55% nonsurgical.

In terms of which experiences were identified as painful and which were identified as producing discomfort, there was wide variation among the patients. The event for which there was most agreement that it was painful was slamming a finger in the door. Ninety-six percent of the patients identified this as painful and 4% as uncomfortable. The highest agreement among patients in terms of what constituted discomfort was itching. Eighty percent of those who had experienced it defined it as producing discomfort, 7% defined it as painful, and 13% said it was neither.

Using 50% as an arbitrary cutoff point, Table 3 summarizes those experiences which 50% or more of the patients defined as painful or as producing discomfort. Those experiences characterized as painful are listed in decreasing order: slamming a finger in a door, a throbbing headache, a sharp sensation in the chest, incisional pain in the first few days postoperatively, muscle cramps or spasms, incisional pain related to coughing the first few days postoperatively, and incisional pain related to getting in and out of bed the first few days postoperatively. Those experiences defined by a majority as producing discomfort were: itching, being in one position for a prolonged period of time, insertion of rubber/plastic tubing through the nose, not being able to drink liquids, feeling of fullness in the abdomen, nausea and vomiting, dull headache, lack of kindness/consideration on the part of care-takers, frequent or continuous shortness of breath, muscle aches, insertion of rubber/plastic tube through rectum, limitation of physical activity, sore throat, and waiting for a new test or procedure to be done. As is apparent, those experiences defined as painful included primarily sharp, throbbing, or acute physical sensations. In contrast, the experiences defined as producing discomfort included psychosocial situations, such as lack of kindness on the part of caretakers or waiting for new test or procedures to be done. Sensations defined as producing discomfort generally were those producing pressure or associated with dullness or aching.

It is clear that there is a great deal of variation in what patients define as painful or as producing discomfort. A major implication of this is that patients must be carefully questioned regarding what they are experiencing. To question a patient only about his pain may not elicit descriptions of other unpleasant sensations or situations he may be experiencing, and comfort measures may be unnecessarily withheld.

In addition to identifying particular experiences as painful or uncomfortable patients were asked to indicate on a ten-point scale how much pain and discomfort they were currently experiencing and what was the worst they had ever experienced. In general, females rated the pain and discomfort they were currently experiencing (4.52 and 4.28) as lower than did males (4.66 and 4.46). When recalling the most severe pain and discomfort they had ever experienced, however, women tended to rate the intensity as higher (9.23 and 9.17) than did men (9.05 and 8.2). That is, women recalled having experienced more severe pain and discomfort than men, but rated their current experiences as lower than the men did. This *may* be related to the nature of experiences defined by men and women as being the worst they had ever experienced. The three experiences identified by men most frequently as being among the worst they had experienced were surgery, fractures and dislocations, and other traumatic events. The experiences indicated by women as producing the most pain were childbirth, surgery, and cramps and spasms. Two of those three

Table 3. Ranking by 200 Patients of Conditions and Procedures as Associated with Pain or Discomfort

Condition or Procedure	N who had experienced	% Identifying as Pain	Condition or Procedure	N who had experienced	% Identifying as Discomfort
Slam finger in door	129	96	Itching	148	80
Headache: throbbing	135	78	Being in one position for prolonged period of time	157	78
Sharp sensation in chest	98	71	Insertion of rubber/plastic tube through nose	83	77
Incision: turning first few days post-op	127	70	Not being able to drink liquids	144	72
Muscle cramps or spasms	155	66	Feeling of Fullness in Abdomen	144	72
Incision: coughing first few days post-op	124	64	Nausea and vomiting	174	70
Incision: getting in/out of bed first few days post-op	126	56	Headache: dull	150	69
			Lack of kindness/consideration on part of care-takers	75	64
			Shortness of breath frequently or continuously	107	63
			Muscle aches	152	63
			Insertion of rubber/plastic tube through rectum	96	57
			Limitation in physical activity	179	55
			Sore throat	169	55
			Waiting for a new test or procedure that will be done to you	173	51

categories are sex related. In summary, women tended to identify different experiences as having produced the worst pain possible and recalled that pain as being worse than pain experiences recalled by men. In contrast, women reported the pain they were currently experiencing to be lower than what the men reported.

The above two sets of patient data illustrate several major points. One is the wide variation in how people define what is ostensibly the same experience or situation. A second point is that, whether patients are feeling pain or discomfort, they may not reflect what they are feeling in either their verbal or nonverbal behavior. This may be because they are not able to accurately interpret and describe what they are experiencing or that, for one reason or another, they try to conceal what they are experiencing. These data were derived from patient samples. Another source of data was from nurses as they attempted to assess patients' pain; the next section of this presentation will report on those data.

PAIN FROM THE NURSE'S POINT OF VIEW

Before presenting the data from nurses, I'd like to mention the work of several other researchers whose observations are relevant to our study of nurses' problems with pain assessment. An earlier quote from Hackett suggested that one problem that exists in terms of assessment of pain is that patients experiencing chronic pain are expected to display the same behaviors as those experiencing acute pain. This was an observation made by Hackett as one of several prejudices that he identified as characterizing physicians, but which may apply equally to nurses. A second prejudice of health professionals identified by Hackett (6) is that in order to hurt, pain must have an organic basis.

Following the tradition of Virchow, we must see cellular pathology before we trust the symptoms. In other words the cell is more reliable than the person. While I would not claim this to be untrue in all cases, it is in many. Furthermore, in practical terms what this means is that the person with a tension headache doesn't suffer as much pain as the man with a brain tumor. In point of fact we have no basis for this distinction because as yet there is no instrument or test that can be used to objectively rate the degree of an individual's pain. The experience of pain is subject to wide alterations even with the same individual.

A third bias described by Hackett has to do with health professionals' tendency to undermedicate patients because of an often unreasonable concern for iatrogenic addiction. Hackett notes that in treating 230 chronically ill patients for whom pain was the principal symptom, only 8 became addicted. He suggests that health professionals are unnecessarily conservative in their use of narcotics to reduce pain. His assertion was substantiated in our observations of patients, particularly oncology patients.

There is some evidence that various health professionals assess the intensity of patients' pain differently. A study by Baer et al. found that of three groups of health professionals, social workers tended to infer that patients have the greatest degree of pain while physicians and nurses inferred less pain (2). The author speculated that persons who have constant contact with patients in pain may feel so overwhelmed by the person's pain that they protect themselves by denying it, or that the health professionals become so familiar with pain that they tune it out.

Another problem is apparent when health professionals and patients vary in assessing the intensity of pain. Wiener (11), in a study of patients experiencing low back pain, noted a number of problems when hospital staff acknowledged the existence of pain but disagreed in terms of the amount of pain. She suggested that the discrepant perspectives related in part to staff inability to diagnose low back pain accurately and to problems in lack of signs of visibility of pain. There is great ambiguity surrounding low back pain, which results in conflicting assessments, with the need for patients to try to legitimize their pain.

In a discussion of pain expression on a burn care unit (4), Fagerhaugh found that staff generally tended to assess pain as less severe than the patient indicated it was, with staff believing that the expression of pain came largely from anxiety. She noted that more experienced nurses tended to use smaller doses of drugs to control pain than did less experienced nurses.

As time went on, nurses gave smaller amounts of drugs and were less concerned with inflicting pain, because they knew the treatments were crucial for recovery. In fact, some nurses can become so inured to pain that they may hum while giving a painful tubbing, much as they might while engaged in any other serious, but not crisis laden, work.

Copp (3), reporting on a study of hospitalized patients, observed that patients who tried various methods to relieve pain at home were reluctant to try such methods while in the hospital because they were afraid that their coping behaviors might be "against the rules" or "might be laughed at as not scientific." She commented that many patients seemed quite able to manage their pain in their own homes, but were at a loss to know how to cope with pain in a hospital.

The problems described by these authors may not be due to any intentional act of omission or commission on the part of nurses, but simply to the fact that we do not know enough about pain assessment and have not given sufficient attention to teaching nurses about it.

In a study done by us at the University of Iowa, of 443 registered and student nurses, subjects were asked to describe one patient situation in which it was difficult to assess pain and one in which it was easy to assess pain. A total of 46 patient behaviors were identified in the analysis of the critical incidents. In general, nurses reported that physiological signs and behaviors were easier indexes to use in pain assessment than was verbal communication. Table 4 shows the percent of responses of various categories. Interestingly enough, in spite of the fact that the single most reliable indicator of how much pain a person is experiencing is the subject's verbal report, verbal communication was fifth in a list of seven categories reflecting various ways of indicating patients' pain. That is, nurses tended to rely more on physiological signs, body movements, facial expressions, and so forth rather than on patients' verbal complaints of pain.

An additional finding of this study was the major problem that exists when the verbal behavior disagrees with the nonverbal behavior presented. This supports the point made by Fordyce and mentioned earlier. In our study, the category of inconsistent verbal and nonverbal behaviors was one of the most frequently used. Interestingly, the category in which assessment was difficult because the person said he was in pain but his nonverbal behavior did not agree was used almost exclusively by the registered nurses. In contrast, the category in which the patient looked as though he was in pain but denied it, was used almost exclusively by student nurses. The registered nurses' concern that they be able to see evidence of pain supports Hackett's assertion that for health professionals, the cell is more reliable than the person.

The problem with the nurses' difficulty in assessing pain has several dimensions. One is that we do not yet know enough about how pain is experienced by patients. A second problem is the wide variation in how pain is experienced and reported by people, and a third is that nurses and other health professionals may gradually become less sensitive to patients' complaints of pain, particularly if they are in a situation where the pain is difficult to alleviate. In the remainder of this chapter, some suggestions will be made regarding what we may do to improve our ability to assess patients' pain.

TOWARD IMPROVEMENT IN ASSESSMENT OF PATIENTS' PAIN

A first step is to try to get better descriptions of what constitutes an average course of pain for patients experiencing different conditions or treatments. One particularly difficult problem in trying to evaluate how much pain patients were having in relation to how much pain patients generally had, was that there are few such descriptions in the literature. We do not even know, for example, the peak periods of pain for patients undergoing many surgical procedures. We need careful and detailed descriptions of patterns of pain and other discomforts commonly experienced by patients.

A second suggestion is the need to be more careful in how we question people about what they are experiencing. If we use the term pain to mean one thing, while a patient is interpreting it to mean something else, we have a classic miscommunication. If a patient responds no to a query about pain, it is not sufficient to leave it there. We should use terms such as discomfort, hurt, sore, ache, pressure, and so forth to try to determine what a patient is experiencing and what we might do to alleviate various unpleasant sensations and conditions.

Table 4. Categories of Cues Used by Nurses in Pain Assessment

Behavior	% of Responses Identified Under "Difficult"	% of Responses Identified Under "Easy"
1. Characteristic of affect or disposition	46	54
2. Oral expression, excluding verbal complaints	35	65
3. Verbal communication	44	56
4. Facial expressions	21	79
5. Body movements	22	78
6. Vital sign changes	22	78
7. Other physiological signs	20	80

Reproduced from Johnson, Assessment of clinical pain, in *Pain: A Sourcebook for Nurses and other Health Professionals.* Ada Jacox, ed. Little, Brown & Co., Boston, 1977, p. 161.

Related to this point is a comment by Fagerhaugh (4), who suggested that, in describing what a patient says about his pain, it may help to use the term patient "reports" pain, as such and such, rather than patient "complains of" pain. The term "complain" has negative connotations for many people and the use of the term "report" may help to neutralize the negativism when it exists.

An examination of one's own attitudes toward pain and what is expected of oneself, and perhaps therefore of others, would also be useful to nurses. Careful attention to what the person who is experiencing the pain is feeling, while trying to minimize one's own beliefs about how pain should be tolerated, may help to make the assessment more subjective.

Related to the problem of learning what a patient is feeling is the need to learn how he usually copes with pain and discomfort if he experiences them at home. As noted earlier, Copp observed that the patients believed the strategies that they used to cope with pain and suffering in their homes may not be acceptable to hospital staff because of their "nonscientific" nature. We need to enlist the patient's assistance both in assessing his condition and in exploring methods of alleviation.

Another focus for concern in improving nurses' ability to assess pain is in teaching nurses to be empathetic and sensitive in eliciting pain descriptions from patients. We probably accept the notion that we ought to teach student nurses, in whatever ways we can, to evaluate patients' pain. Perhaps even more important, however, is that those nurses who have been in practice for sometime become resensitized to the need for careful pain assessments. It is too easy to slip into an acceptance of the familiar, and when one works for days, weeks, and years with patients in pain, one may well tend to become immune to expressions of pain. We need to reassess our own assessment abilities periodically in a conscious and deliberate way.

Finally, to end on the same note on which I began, I would like to emphasize that probably the most useful thing nurses can do in trying to assess patients' pain is to remember that pain is a subjective phenomenon and if we are to understand it, we must not only observe the person's behavior, but must listen to what the one who is experiencing it says about it.

ACKNOWLEDGMENT

This chapter incorporates the findings of research supported by DHEW, Division of Nursing, from 1970-1976, by Grants NU-00387 and NU-00467.

REFERENCES

1. Abrams, R.D. The patient with cancer—his changing pattern of communication. *N. Eng. J. Med.* 274, 317-322, (1966).
2. Baer, E., Davitz, L.J., and Lieb, R. Inferences of physical pain and psychological distress: 1. In relation to verbal and nonverbal patient communication. *Nurs. Res.* 5, 388-401 (1970).
3. Copp, L.A. The spectrum of suffering. *Am. J. Nurs.* 3, 491-495 (1974).
4. Fagerhaugh, S.Y. Pain expression and control on a burn care unit. *Nurs. Outlook* 10, 645-650 (1974).
5. Fordyce, W.E. *Behavioral Methods for Chronic Pain and Illness.* C.V. Mosby, St. Louis, 1976, pp. 11-25.
6. Hackett, T.P. Pain and prejudice: Why do we doubt that the patient is in pain? *Med. Times* 2, 130-141 (1971).
7. Hardy, J.D. The nature of pain. *J. Chron. Dis.* 7, 22-51 (1956).
8. Hilgard, E. Pain as a puzzle for psychology and physiology. *Am. Psychol.* 103-113 (1969).
9. Jacox, A. and Stewart, M. *Psychosocial Contingencies of the Pain Experience.* univ. of Iowa College of Nursing, Iowa City, 1973.
10. Sternbach, R.A. *Pain: A Psychophysiological Analysis.* Academic Press, New York, 1968.
11. Wiener, C.L. Pain assessment on an orthopedic ward. *Nurs. Outlook* 8, 508-516 (1975).

CHAPTER 6

Clinical Pharmacology of Pain

S. GEORGE CARRUTHERS

Alleviation of pain by pharmacological means is a time-honored attribute of the healing professions. There are many more interesting, elaborate, and even satisfying therapeutic interventions, but seldom is the sense of patient relief or gratitude so great as when a particularly severe or persistent pain is abolished. This knowledge creates a very real temptation for the clinician to fail to diagnose precisely or to consider adequately the pathophysiological processes involved, to ignore the sociopsychological factors such as fear and anxiety, or to underestimate the role of the patient-physician relationship, by adopting a simple empirical approach and by prescribing unnecessarily excessive or powerful analgesics.

Therapeutic skills in pain relief require the application of the same principles as any other form of treatment (4):

What is the basic diagnosis?
What are the defects in normal physiology?
What is the rational drug (or nondrug) therapy?
What can reasonably be expected from drugs, considering the natural progression, remission, and variation of the disease?
How will improvement be assessed: subjectively by the patient, subjectively by the clinician, or by objective measurements?

How long will treatment be pursued: an acute crisis, a chronic disorder, lifetime maintenance?

What is the appropriate dose of medication, considering the nature and severity of disease, intercurrent illness, age and weight?

What are the potential problems with the medication(s): adverse effects, interactions with concurrent medications for other disorders, including nonprescription medicines and social drugs, in particular alcohol?

WHAT IS THE BASIC DIAGNOSIS?

The role of precise diagnosis cannot be overstated. Symptomatic relief of pain plays an important role in the early management of many conditions, both medical and surgical. The therapeutic maxim of "No treatment before diagnosis" should be observed strictly if symptomatic measures are likely to obscure important physical signs. This applies particularly to the painful abdomen, the result of visceral inflammation, ulceration or infarction, for which the correct intervention may be delayed if physical signs are masked.

Serious diagnostic hazards include the misinterpretation of headache due to leaking cerebral artery aneurysm, failure to recognize the cause of postoperative "muscle cramps" as deep venous thrombosis, and misconstruing intussusception as simple colic in a baby. To interpret a painful toe as a result of local trauma may be a disservice to the gouty patient by failing to provide appropriate therapy, but also by aggravating the condition if usual analgesic doses of aspirin are prescribed, thereby enhancing urate retention.

WHAT ARE THE DEFECTS IN NORMAL PHYSIOLOGY?

The inflammatory process concerned with pain is associated with release of prostaglandins, leukocyte migration and discharge of factors such as histamine, and damage to lysosomal membranes causing release of injurious enzymes. One or all of these processes may occur in a given painful situation. The background activity of endorphins, natural morphine-like substances, may influence an individual's responsiveness to the painful stimulus. The common nervous pathway for pain appreciation involves the transmission of impulses by small unmyelinated C fibers and by the delta group of A fibers in afferent neurons, the lateral spinothalamic tract, the thalamus, and the sensory cortex of the postcentral gyrus. Pain may be pharmacologically altered at each of these levels (9). The most rational approach is to alter or remove the provoking abnormality. If that approach is not feasible, peripheral alteration at the pain ending by simple analgesic drugs, by local anesthetic action on the nerve endings, peripheral nerve, nerve plexus, or nerve roots, by chemical or surgical destruction of the spinothalamic tract or by central alteration of pain by strong analgesics, anesthetics, tranquilizers, sedatives, and hypnotics can all be considered.

Table 1. Painful Disorders Treated With Drugs
Which Are Not Conventionally Accepted As Analgesics

Disease State	Drug(s)

Angina pectoris	nitrites, e.g.,
	   nitroglycerine
	   isosorbide dinitrate
	 β-blockers, e.g.,
	   propranolol
	   metoprololol
	   timololol

Gout	allopurinol probenicid sulfinpyrazone colchicine
Migraine	ergotamine
Trigeminal neuralgia	carbamazepine
Glaucoma	carbonic anhydrase inhibitors, e.g., acetazolamide
Giant cell arteritis	corticosteroids
Peptic ulcer	antacids carbenoxolone cimetidine
Aortic dissection	β-blockers reserpine
Infective disorders	appropriate antibiotics
Paget's disease	calcitonin mithramycin editronate sodium

Table 1 illustrates some disorders in which knowledge of the pathophysiology has led to pain control by drugs which are not considered analgesic in the classical sense. The genesis of gout is the deposition of urate crystals in joint synovium, with subsequent leukocyte phagocytosis and the release from the leukocytes of substances which initiate the pain response. Urate concentration may be reduced by dietary alteration, prevention of excessive cellular breakdown, and reduction of diuretics and other drugs which impair renal elimination of urate. Leukocyte migration and degradation might be prevented. Nonspecific efforts at altering the production of the prostaglandins and other substances which irritate the nerve endings might be undertaken. In clinical practice, the relief of gouty pain may involve one or more of these approaches. Allopurinol competitively inhibits xanthin-oxidase, preventing the transformation of soluble hypoxanthine to the relatively insoluble uric acid. Colchicine alters the leukocyte response and probenicid or sulfinpyrazone may be administered for their uricosuric effects. Prostaglandin biosynthesis is inhibited and lysosome membrane is stablized by phenylbutazone, which exerts antiinflammatory and analgesic effects important in the early stages of management before other measures are effective.

The same principles may be applied to the other conditions listed in Table 1. Angina pectoris is the direct result of a relative deficiency of oxygen in the myocardium. Factors contributing to this oxygen deficit at a given workload include left ventricular size and force of contraction, systolic blood pressure, and heart rate. The nitrites reduce cardiac preload and afterload and tend to reduce heart size, but provoke reflex tachycardia. Beta-blockers such as propranolol reduce systolic blood pressure and heart rate, but tend to increase oxygen consumption by a direct negative inotropic effect which increases heart size. By interfering with sympathetic drive to the myocardium, beta-blockers may even promote frank congestive heart failure. A drug in either group or a combination may be effective in reducing or eliminating the pain of angina, providing their limitations are recognized.

Many painful conditions are the result of bacterial infection. Appropriate and adequate antimicrobial therapy is the single most important therapeutic measure in conditions such as sinusitis, cholecystitis, and pyelonephritis, but it would hardly be considered good practice to ignore the patient's pain while the effect of the antibiotic or surgical drainage were awaited.

WHAT IS THE RATIONAL DRUG (OR NONDRUG) THERAPY?

Only drug therapy will be considered, since other aspects of analgesia (psychotherapy, acupuncture, biofeedback) have been considered elsewhere. The choice of appropriate analgesia rests between four major groups of drugs defined by common usage as (a) strong analgesics, (b) mild or weak analgesics, (c) antiinflammatory drugs, and (d) psychotropic drugs. Since the members of these groups are well known to most clinicians, only specific aspects will be discussed in detail.

Strong Analgesics

This group consists of opium extracts of variable purity, pure natural alkaloid derivatives of opium, such as morphine, semisynthetic pharmaceutical preparations of morphine, such as oxycodone, and totally synthetic pharmaceutical preparations which have structural and pharmacological similarity to morphine, such as methadone. The strong analgesics are essentially synonymous with narcotic analgesics except for two substances which are considered neither as powerful nor potentially addictive, pentazocine and methotrimeprazine. The other drugs are subject to strict national and international regulations to prevent their abuse. The narcotic analgesics differ in potency and in their ability to cause adverse effects, but appear to be relatively similar in their efficacy and are more powerful than the nonnarcotic analgesics.

The narcotic analgesics also differ in terms of pharmaceutical purity, although that is rarely a problem when the pure alkaloids, semisynthetics or synthetic preparations are used. Pharmacological considerations include systemic bioavailability which will be discussed further under First Pass Effect, rate of onset of effect, rate of drug elimination, and duration of activity. The drugs appear to differ in their potential for tolerance and dependence, but the factors influencing this are related as much to availability on the street and poorly understood psychological aspects of addiction, as to pharmacological considerations.

Morphine is the strong analgesic of choice for most physicians, although others may prefer meperidine, levorphanol, or methadone. In Britain the legitimate use of heroin is highly favored.

Strong analgesics play a major role in the management of visceral pain. This includes myocardial infarction, gastrointestinal colic, biliary colic, ureteric colic, and the pain associated with childbirth. The pharmacological effect appears to be mediated by stimulation of enkephalin receptors in the central nervous system. The central analgesic effect is often accompanied by a feeling of enhanced well being or euphoria, occasionally drowsiness and mental clouding. The medullary cough center is directly suppressed, the sensitivity of the respiratory center to carbon dioxide is diminished, causing respiratory depression, and nausea or vomiting are provoked by direct stimulation of the chemoreceptor trigger zone. Tolerance and dependence are discussed later. Stimulation of enkephalin receptors in the gastrointestinal tract may be partly responsible for the common effects of constipation, while direct smooth muscle activity may provoke spasm of the sphincter of Oddi or the ureters, aggravating biliary and ureteric colic, respectively. Pupillary meiosis and hypoventilation limit the use of the narcotics in head injury and respiratory depression, respectively. Nausea and vomiting often require symptomatic management and many physicians undertake prophylaxis by prescribing antiemetics, such as cyclizine, dimenhydrinate, and prochlorperazine, to avoid further distress to the patient.

Only approximately 20% of an oral dose of morphine reaches the systemic circulation (7). First pass metabolism in the liver appears to be important. Parenteral (intramuscular or intravenous) administration is therefore preferred. Onset of action is rapid, essentially at once following intravenous (iv) doses, permitting simple control of therapeutic and adverse effects, and within half an hour following intramuscular (im) and subcutaneous injection, which permit the clinician less direct control of pain relief and nausea. Morphine is almost entirely metabolized in the liver. Individuals with liver disease appear to be at enhanced risk of adverse effects. Not only is morphine eliminated more slowly than the usual half-life of 2 to 2½ hr, but cerebral "sensitivity" to morphine may be enhanced with possible precipitation of hepatic encephalopathy.

Mild Analgesics

These are less effective than narcotic analgesics in relieving pain. They are usually ineffective in relieving severe pain of any sort, especially that arising from surgery, bone fracture or the visceral disorders discussed earlier. Late postoperative pain, dysmenorrhea, toothache, headache, and moderately severe musculoskeletal pain, are pain disorders frequently treated with this group of analgesics. Some members have additional antipyretic and antiinflammatory properties. The latter group is described in more detail later.

Chemically, the agents in this subgroup are diverse. A few are structurally related to the narcotics, including codeine, dihydrocodeine, and propoxyphene. The salicylate group include acetylsalicylic acid (ASA, aspirin), sodium salicylate, and salicylamide. The para-aminophenol derivatives include acetaminophen and phenacetin. The pyrazolone derivatives include aminopyrine and dipyrone whose use has been curtailed by serious hematological effects. The related drugs, phenylbutazone and oxyphenbutazone, are discussed with the antiinflammatory agents, while another member of the family, sulfinpyrazone, although devoid of analgesic effect, is discussed in the treatment of gout.

Salicylates are the cornerstone of most antipyretic, mild analgesic, or antiinflammatory regimens. Their important role in the management of arthritis places them clearly with the antiinflammatory drugs with which they will be discussed.

Acetaminophen is in fact a metabolite of phenacetin but does not appear to have the potential for renal damage of its parent. Earlier members of the family, derivatives of aniline, are no longer used because of hematological toxicity. The drugs are devoid of central effect, exerting their analgesic effects peripherally. Acetaminophen has certain advantages over aspirin. It has little effect on coagulation, is not associated with gastric irritation (apart from occasional overdoses) and is not known to cause asthma or nasal polyps. Indeed, toxicity is remarkably uncommon, but serious hepatic necrosis and death have occurred after large overdoses. The proposed mechanism is interesting and bears repetition. The usual metabolism of acetaminophen involves the formation of conjugates with glucuronide or sulfate, thus a minor, but potentially harmful, oxidative metabolite is rendered inert by binding with glutathione (12). Excessive doses of acetaminophen, particularly in individuals with induced oxidative metabolism, e.g., alcohol or barbiturate users, or a relative deficiency of hepatic glutathione reserves, e.g., malnutrition, produce increased amounts of the hepatotoxic metabolite which binds covalently with liver cells. There has been considerable interest in the early management of acetaminophen overdosage with surrogates of endogenous glutathione, such as cysteamine and acetylcysteine (13).

Codeine is 3-0-methyl morphine and it differs from morphine mainly in terms of potency as well as efficacy. Indeed, about 10% of all the administered codeine is transformed in the liver by demethylation of morphine. Unlike the majority of the narcotics, codeine is effective orally, with the maximum effect in 1 to 2 hr after administration. Large doses have the same serious adverse effects as the narcotics.

Propoxyphene is structurally related to methadone and differs like codeine from the narcotics in terms of efficacy and potency. Propoxyphene and codeine have both been associated with dependence and abuse. Overdose effects of both are reversible by morphine antagonists such as naloxone. Neither drug has been shown to be significantly more efficacious than the salicylates. Their frequent casual use must therefore be viewed with some concern.

Antiinflammatory Drugs

This group of analgesics encompasses the family which is otherwise known as antirheumatic agents. One of the cardinal aims of treatment of rheumatic disease is the reduction of inflammatory change, with reduction of joint pain and stiffness, improved mobility and diminished disability. Narcotic analgesics without antiinflammatory properties have little role to play in reducing the pain of rheumatic diseases. Although they may relieve pain, their use must be criticized on the grounds that they fail to reduce underlying inflammation and, possibly by blunting the patient's protective defences, might even lead to further joint destruction.

Aspirin remains the cardinal member of this group, yet its important effects are often underutilized. Large near-toxic doses of salicylates are often required to exert antiinflammatory effects. At these doses and associated plasma concentrations, many patients experience gastrointestinal disturbance. Physicians are sometimes reluctant and patients sometimes unwilling to take the numerous pills required. Thoughtlessly, some clinicians go first to the newer, much more expensive nonsteroidal antiinflammatory agents whose gastric irritant properties may be less, although not always so. A more rational approach is the use of microfined and enteric coated salicylate preparations, in gradually increasing doses, using the available large 10 grain (650 mg) tablets. If there are contraindications to the use of aspirin, if toxicity occurs, or if the maximum desirable therapeutic effect is not achieved on salicylates alone at near-toxic doses, progression to the other agents is the next reasonable step. It is a sad fact that further remedies are more likely to be accompanied by increasingly serious adverse effects.

Phenylpropionic acid derivatives such as ibuprofen and fenoprofen have antiinflammatory analgesic and antipyretic properties and like their near relative, naproxen, are effective adjunctive therapy in many patients with rheumatic diseases.

Phenylbutazone and oxyphenylbutazone are pyrazolone derivatives with analgesic, antiinflammatory, and antipyretic properties. Like the only other clinically available member of their family, sulfinpyrazone, they also have uricosuric activity. They appear like other antiinflammatory agents to inhibit prostaglandin synthetase and to stabilize lysosome membrane. Their highly predictable efficacy encourages their widespread and often excessive use. Appropriate benefit/risk ratios are encountered in the management of ankylosing spondylitis and acute attacks of gout. Otherwise, risk generally outweighs benefit. Their use in conditions where adequate trials of aspirin or other antiinflammatory or analgesic agents has not first been attempted is to be deplored. It is an unfortunate consequence of clinical practice that the most devastating adverse effects of drugs seem to occur most frequently in those patients where their use may not have been fully justified.

Indomethacin, which acts by inhibiting prostaglandin E_2, is an important reserve agent with the advantage of a suppository preparation, permitting evening dosage and reduced morning stiffness. Unfortunately, indomethacin suffers from an extremely high incidence of adverse effects.

Psychotropic Drugs

The mood altering properties of the narcotic analgesics has been mentioned. There are many other drugs which influence the response to pain, even though they are totally devoid of analgesic activity. Historically, alcohol has played an important role in the management of operative and postoperative pain in both military and civilian surgical procedures in the pre-anaesthetic era. Today, we rely on major tranquilizers, such as chlorpromazine, a phenothiazine, and haloperidol, a butyrophenone. The mood altering properties of cocaine are exploited in the popular Brompton cocktail. The need for these drugs arises mainly in the management of patients with chronic, intractable pain, either alone or in combination with various surgical approaches. These are usually patients with terminal cancer, in whom addiction is not a concern, but in whom a high quality of residual life is desirable. Adequate use of nonnarcotic analgesics should not be overlooked. A comprehensive review of this topic is not possible here, but interested readers are recommended to study Chapter 2 in this volume as well as the articles by Kubler-Ross et al. and Liegner.

WHAT CAN REASONABLY BE EXPECTED FROM DRUGS?

The patient's answer to this question is simple and clear—complete and continuous relief of pain! While that is highly idealistic, it is more realistic to warn the patient that he may have to tolerate some pain from time to time in the interest of avoiding potentially addicting drugs or unduly large doses of drugs which are predictably likely to alter his ability to function well or to cause serious adverse effects. With these thoughts in mind, patients must then be assessed on an individual basis. It is patently cruel to deny adequate analgesia to a patient whose severe back pain is caused by a metastatic tumor. The actual cruelty may be less, but the potential for real harm may be greater, if a patient with vague abdominal discomfort receives frequent injections of narcotics without diagnosis or otherwise appropriate management. This creates a heavy responsibility for the clinician primarily involved in a patient's care. A thorough evaluation of the cause of pain and exploration of alternative analgesic measures, perhaps in collaboration with a Pain Clinic, may be desirable.

HOW WOULD IMPROVEMENT BE ASSESSED?

Since pain is a subjective phenomenon, experienced only by the individual who complains of it, subjective responsiveness is the obvious and usual means of assessing efficacy. However, because of the potential for abuse of the narcotics by a small minority of unusually devious patients, the skills of careful objective observers, usually nurses, may be needed when "pain" is unusually prolonged, unduly frequent, unassociated with the usual affective appearance, in pain relieved at an unusually rapid rate (almost, as it were, improved by the sight of a needle), or associated with vague, ill-defined clinical conditions which behoove the unfortunate "sufferer" to attend numerous primary care physicians or emergency departments. Fortunately, the usual patient-physician relationship is based on more honest patient behavior. Neurotic and hysterical individuals who describe pain as a major component of their symptoms often prove not only difficult to evaluate but to treat.

HOW LONG WILL TREATMENT BE PURSUED?

Clinical knowledge of the usual duration of pain in a given situation is a prerequisite to determining the duration of analgesic therapy. The surgeon appreciates that pain sufficiently severe to require narcotic analgesia may persist from 1 to 3 days following appendectomy or cholecystectomy. He realizes that prolonged or excessive narcotic analgesia is likely to depress respiration, increase the likelihood of pulmonary atelectasis, produce or enhance postoperative nausea and vomiting, impair gastrointestinal motility and encourage constipation. While it is in the patient's interest to have adequate analgesia, prolonged treatment is counterproductive. Analgesic management must also be sufficiently flexible to permit the occasional patient with protracted pain adequate analgesia to ambulate, respond to the physiotherapist's demands for active inspiration and forced coughing, or simply to obtain sufficient rest free of pain to facilitate recovery.

Certain chronic conditions, such as ankylosing spondylitis and rheumatoid arthritis, are ultimately self-limiting and may enter a "burnt-out" phase. Analgesia beyond this stage is without benefit, but potential hazards persist. Rational management requires thorough knowledge of the natural history of disease, clinical appreciation of improvement or resolution and simple empirical attempts at reduction or discontinuation of therapy to evaluate response.

It is likely that most patients requiring analgesia of the Brompton cocktail type will continue for life on such medications and may, indeed, require intermittent parenteral doses of narcotics during periods of crisis. The patient with gout will likewise carry his need for continuous prophylaxis and intermittent acute management to the grave. In both circumstances, it would generally be foolhardy to discontinue treatment once its need had been clearly demonstrated.

WHAT IS THE APPROPRIATE DOSE?

The therapeutic aphorism that the therapeutic dose of an analgesic is enough is an effective approach to dosage considerations. Since pain is subjective, it occurs in all degrees of severity and is influenced by a large number of biological factors. A blanket approach is therefore unsatisfactory. The clinician should start with the dose which is usually appropriate to the disease state, disease severity, age, weight, and intercurrent disease status of the patient. If the therapeutic objective is achieved without adverse effect, the dose may be maintained, but if not, gradual adjustments are necessary until either the goal of pain relief occurs or unwanted effects develop. If no benefit is achieved, an unrelated analgesic of the same or a more powerful group may be administered. The physician must ensure that he is not dealing with a condition more appropriately relieved by other means (Table 1). The use of ancillary techniques such as splinting, bed rest, traction, antibiotics, local radiotherapy, the relief of depression or the creation of mild euphoria should not be overlooked.

WHAT ARE THE POTENTIAL PROBLEMS?

It is not possible in this short space to recount the numerous adverse effects. Some more important toxic effects have been mentioned in passing. A comprehensive, albeit unweighted, list of adverse reactions is easily obtained in the product monograph. Some of the more common or significant adverse reactions associated with individual drugs are listed in Table 2.

A modern pharmacological review of analgesia would be incomplete without some mention of endorphins, enkephalins, narcotic antagonists, tolerance and dependence. First past effect and placebo activity are other topics which merit brief discussion.

PHYSIOLOGICAL MORPHINE-LIKE SUBSTANCES AND RECEPTORS

Stereochemical studies with morphine indicate that there are specific receptor sites in several parts of the brain and, indeed, even in the gastrointestinal tract which act as specific sites for the action of morphine and other narcotic analgesics (14). There is increasing evidence for endogenous morphine-like substances in both the brain and pituitary which bind with narcotic antagonists. The endogenous morphines or "endorphins" include substances known as "enkephalins" and are thought to act as natural analgesics at specific subcellular binding sites. The exact role played by these

Table 2. Common Adverse Effects of Analgesics

Analgesics	Effects
Strong	
Morphine	nausea, vomiting, constipation,
Heroin ⁄	dizziness, confusion, hallucination,
Oxycodone	respiratory depression,
Meperidine	pulmonary edema,
Methadone	tolerance, dependence,
Methotrimeprazine	increased pulmonary resistance,
Pentazocine	respiratory failure
Mild	
Acetaminophen (a)	analgesic nephropathy (b)
Phenacetin (b)	renal failure, hepatic failure (a)
	cardiorespiratory failure
Propoxyphene	see Strong Analgesics
Codeine	
Salicylates	see below
Antiinflammatory	
Salicylates	nausea, vomiting, dyspepsia, gastrointestinal hemorrhage, tinnitus, hearing loss, rash, asthma, nose polyps, prolonged prothrombin time, platelet aggregation impaired (ASA), metabolic acidosis, respiratory alkalosis, cardiovascular collapse
Ibuprofen	nausea, vomiting, dyspepsia,
Fenprofen	gastrointestinal hemorrhage,
Naproxen	drowsiness, dizziness, headache,
Tolmetin	fluid retention, edema,
Indomethacin	marrow suppresion (c),
Phenylbutazone (c)	variable effects on prothrombin time and platelets,
Oxyphenbutazone (c)	hypersensitivity reactions

(a), (b), (c) Indicate that a particular adverse effect is more common with the individual analgesics indicated.

substances in an individual's responsiveness to pain remains uncertain.

Until the development of naloxone, previous narcotic antagonists such as nalorphine were capable also of exerting some morphine-like activity and were said to have "partial agonist" activity. Naloxone appears to be a pure antagonist, which, even when given in large quantities, does not exert analgesic or other central morphine-like effects. The distinction by the body of such trivial differences in chemical structure is strong supporting evidence for a specific cellular receptor for the narcotics. Naloxone is effective against overdose from all the morphine-related drugs and may be given safely to other comatose patients with small pupils in whom the diagnosis of narcotic overdose is only slightly suspected.

TOLERANCE AND DEPENDENCE

Tolerance is the phenomenon of increasing dosage requirements in patients who receive narcotic analgesics over a prolonged period of time. The phenomenon is thought not to be a pharmacokinetic one, but a change in receptor responsiveness. There is no evidence that the plasma concentrations of the narcotics become any less with continued dosing or that changes in protein binding occur, but rather that the same amounts of analgesic are available and produce a diminished effect with time. Dependence is quite a different phenomenon. It may be preceded by tolerance, but it is complicated by social and psychological factors which are not well understood. The behavioral aspects may relate to the "high" feelings associated with the narcotics. It is quite common for patients who require prolonged analgesia with the narcotics to demonstrate little evidence of dependence while others, with both appropriate and inappropriate motivations for their initial use of narcotics, become addicted with relative ease. A more thorough appreciation of the role of the endogenous morphines and their specific receptor sites may help us understand better the phenomenon of tolerance and dependence.

FIRST PASS EFFECT

It is a simple clinical observation that certain narcotic analgesics appear ineffective when taken orally, while others appear equally effective whether given by similar oral or parenteral dosage. It might be suspected that such differences are due simply to absorption from the gastrointestinal tract, but such is generally not the case. Studies involving radio labeled drugs demonstrate that similar excretion of radioactivity occurs whether the drug is given orally or parenterally. The essential difference then is what happens to the drug during its absorptive phase, in passing through the gastrointestinal tract and the liver before entering the systemic circulation. The fraction of drug which reaches this systemic circulation is often known as that which is "systemically available" and the destruction of parent drug on passage through the gut or liver as the "first pass effect" (4). A very interesting practical application of this phenomenon occurs in the utilization of a combination of methadone and the specific narcotic antagonist naloxone in the management of heroin addicts (8). Methadone has a prolonged duration of action and is suitable for once daily dosage. It is well absorbed from the oral route, but absorption is sufficiently slow so that the peak concentration in plasma is attentuated and a "high" is avoided. Naloxone essentially undergoes total hepatic metabolism during the first pass and therefore exerts no narcotic antagonist effect when taken orally in combination with methadone. Abusers of heroin are well aware that methadone will produce a satisfactory replacement effect if injected iv. Such individuals are well known for their ability to overstate their methadone needs in attempts to have a surplus for later personal abuse or for the street market. However, if methadone with naloxone added is dissolved in water and injected, the naloxone produces an immediate narcotic withdrawal effect. Turning "cold turkey" is not at all desirable for the addict! Variation in the first pass effect is likely to occur when there is significant intrahepatic or extrahepatic shunting from the portal to the systemic circulation, a factor which should be borne in mind when the narcotic addict also has a history of alcohol abuse.

PLACEBO RESPONSE

Satisfactory relief of pain by a placebo was produced in 35% of 1082 patients with a variety of painful conditions ranging from headache to angina pectoris (1). The concept of a placebo "reactor" has also been described by Beecher et al. (2). Reactors, the patients who are responsive to placebo, are thought to have several characteristics, such as extroversion, desire for hospitalization, presence of constipation, and anxiety, but these features are generally too loose to make clear distinctions between individuals. It is generally true, however, that the greater the psychological component of pain, the more likely the placebo is to work. Use of the placebo is charged with problems. The physician feels that he is duping his patient and most patients feel angry and disenchanted if they discover that the medication which they felt was helping them turns out to be nothing more than candy coated sugar. Many physicians interpret a patient's response to placebo as an indication that the patient is in fact hysterical or malingering, while there is in fact no justification for this assumption. For these reasons, the placebo is more often abused than used appropriately and has been the object of serious criticism by Bok (5). For a thorough review of placebo response, the reader is advised to read Bourne (6).

The consideration of placebo is perhaps a pertinent note on which to end this discussion of drugs in analgesia. The physician must remember that his empathy with the patient, his attitude, his supportiveness, as much as the pills which he prescribes or the narcotic analgesics which are injected, play an important role in the relief of the patient's pain and contribute to his therapeutic effectiveness.

REFERENCES

1. Beecher, J.K. The powerful placebo. *J. Am. Med. Assoc.* 159, 1602-1606 (1955).
2. Beecher, H.K., Keats, A.S., Mosteller, F., and Lasagna, L. The effectiveness of oral analgesics (morphine, codeine, acetylsalicylic acid) and the problem of placebo "reactors" and "non-reactors." *J. Pharmacol. Exp. Ther.* 109, 393-400 (1953).
3. Bochner, F., Carruthers, G., Kampmann, J., and Steiner, J. Drug information: A means to improve prescribing, in *Handbook of Clinical Pharmacology.* Little, Brown & Company, Boston, Mass., 1978, ch. 2, pp. 10-19.
4. Bochner, F., Carruthers, G., Kampmann, J. and Steiner, J. Definition of terms, in *Handbook of Clinical Pharmacology.* Little, Brown & Company, Boston, Mass., 1978, ch. 10, pp. 68-85.
5. Bok, S. The ethics of giving placebos. *Sci. Am.* 231, 17-23 (1974).
6. Bourne, H.R. Rational use of placebo, in *Clinical Pharmacology. Basic Principles in Therapeutics.* K.L. Melmon and H.F. Morelli eds. Macmillan, New York, 1978, ch. 24, 1052-1062.
7. Brunk, S.F. and Delle, M. Morphine metabolism in man. *Clin. Pharmacol. Ther.* 16, 51-57, (1974).
8. Dole, V.P. and Nyswander, M.E. A medical treatment for diacetylmorphine (heroin) addiction. *J. Am. Med. Assoc.* 193, 646-650 (1965).
9. Dundee, J.W. and McCaughey, W. Drugs in anaesthetic practice, in *Drug Treatment. Principles and Practice of Clinical Pharmacology and Therapeutics.* G.S. Gary, ed. Publishing Sciences Group Inc., Acton, Mass., 1976, ch. 9, pp. 214-251.
10. Kübler-Ross, E., Wessler, S. and Avioli, L.V. On death and dying. *J. Am. Med. Assoc.* 221, 174 (1972).
11. Liegner, L.M. St. Christopher's Hospice, 1974: Care of the dying patient. *J. Am. Med. Assoc.* 234, 1047 (1975).
12. Mitchell, J.R., Thorgeirsson, S.S., Potter, W.Z. et al. Acetaminophen-induced hepatic injury: Protective role of glutathione in man and rationale for therapy. *Clin. Pharmacol. Ther.* 16, 676-684 (1974).
13. Prescott, L.F., Park, J., and Proudfoot, A.T. Cysteamine for paracetamol poisoning. *Lancet* 1, 357 (1976).
14. Simon, E.J. and Hiller, J.M. The opiate receptors, in *Annual Review of Pharmacology and Toxicology.* R. George, R. Okun, and A.K. Cho, eds. Annual Reviews Inc., Palo Alto, Calif., 1978, ch. 18, pp. 371-394.

CHAPTER 7

Psychological and Psychiatric Aspects of Pain Control

H. MERSKEY

PSYCHIATRIC DIAGNOSIS OF PAIN

The management of almost all patients with pain requires that attention be paid to their psychological state. Some of the evidence concerning this is provided in the discussion on the nature of pain (p. 71), where it was noted that pain is frequently associated with psychiatric illness. Other evidence relates to the fluctuation of pain with mood, which was also discussed. The frequent association of pain with psychiatric disorder is almost certainly due in part to a selection process. It has been shown that only about 3% of all instances of bodily symptoms such as headache, dizziness, and vomiting were reported to family practitioners (1). Thus even if a symptom has a physical basis it is not automatically brought to the attention of physicians. The final decision depends upon attitudes, feelings, and ideas that the individual may have about his complaint. Hence patients with pain are invariably a selected population. Nevertheless it becomes relevant to enquire: Who are the patients who complain of pain?

The first answer is nearly all patients of any sort. If, next, we look at chronic pain there is obviously an enormous variety of potential causes, especially neurological damage and musculoskeletal disorder, but also visceral disturbances and pain from carcinoma involving one or more of the above systems. Low back pain, whether its causes are physical or psychological, is the commonest diagnosis in most pain clinics. Investigation of the psychiatric characteristics of these patients has produced some broad agreement.

Psychiatric patients, selected only for the presence of pain, tend to cover the broad spectrum of affective and neurotic illness. Depression, anxiety, and sometimes complaints with hypochondriacal or hysterical features are all present, with the neurotic end of the spectrum predominating (35). In comparison with those who do not have pain, the proportions with endogenous depression are reduced and those with schizophrenia are low or few. This pattern increases in sharpness when the pain has been present for more than 3 months by comparison with other psychiatric patients also ill for more than 3 months (19). Endogenous depression and schizophrenia have limited or almost no representation among the more chronic pain population, and the bulk consists of patients with anxiety and with hysterical features or hypochondriasis, or a mixture of all three. Some patients have neurotic depression, again with a mixture of anxiety and hysterical features. Among those who are thought to have hysterical syndromes, about half have a past history of conversion symptoms, while another half have evidence of a hysterical personality, and both those with and without conversion symptoms in the past have an excess of somatic symptoms (20).

Among the psychiatric patients with chronic pain there is an increase in the family history of pain (20), an excess of consultations, and sexual disturbance in relative excess of that found in other psychiatric patients (20). Spouses and their relations also have a significant increase in the history of pain (20, 26). The modal pattern of the British psychiatric patient with pain, who is not unlike that described in the American literature, was pictured once as follows: *"A married woman of the working or lower class, possibly once pretty and appealing, but never keen on sexual intercourse, now faded and complaining with a history of repeated negative physical examinations and investigations, frank conversion symptoms in up to 50% of cases in addition to the pain, and a sad tale of a hard life; together with depression which does not respond to antidepressant drugs"* (21).

Psychologists studying pain in North America report findings which correspond to this. Starting with Hanvik (13), the low back pain patient was shown to have the conversion V triad on the Minnesota Multiphasic Personality Inventory (MMPI). That is to say the patients show elevations on the Hysteria and Hypochondriasis scales with a lower intervening elevation on the Depression scale. Reports on patients with back pain (14, 37) and to some extent facial pain (34) confirm these patterns, which correspond psychometrically to the English clinical reports.

Patients in pain clinics in Australia (29) and in Seattle (28) have also been demonstrated to show patterns of "abnormal illness bahvior" similar to that designated conversion reaction or hypochondriacal reaction. This may not be true for the majority of patients in all pain clinics, particularly those much concerned with carcinoma pain or defined neurological syndromes, but it will probably often apply to many of the numerous patients with psychiatric disturbances seen in pain clinics everywhere. These conclusions on diagnosis enable us to consider further the mechanisms by which pain of psychological origin occurs.

MECHANISM OF PAIN

Occasional patients with schizophrenia appear to have hallucinations of pain. This is an extremely rare mechanism, certainly by comparison with the other ways in which pain may occur. However perhaps somewhat more patients among the few with endogenous depression who have pain, experience depressive hallucinations; for example, a patient who had the feeling that she had pains jabbing in her vagina and buttocks and whose pains went away following electroconvulsive therapy (ECT). The most commonly accepted mechanism for pain of psychological origin invokes a physical route. This is the notion of tension pain. It is suggested that muscle contraction gives rise to chronic aching or discomfort or pain, when the waste products of metabolism are not carried away sufficiently fast. The exact physical basis of muscle tension pain is not known, but it undoubtedly occurs.

In anxious patients there is a liability to increased tension. This sets up some pain, the pain may make the anxiety worse and the anxiety may make the tension worse in a vicious circle. This theory is attractive and it has been shown that muscle tension is increased both in relation to anxiety and in muscles which could be related to headache, e.g., frontalis (48). Moreover relaxation, biofeedback, psychotherapy, and anxiolytic drugs, e.g.,Diazepam, relieve much pain supposedly due to tension. Unfortunately, and perhaps inevitably, this is not the whole story. It has not been shown that pain and anxiety are directly related in sufficient proportion to muscle tension to account for the pain. Many patients with pain of psychological origin exist who do not show evidence of muscle tension clinically or respond to the appropriate treatments; and the group of chronic patients with hysterical features is prominent in this respect.

An alternative hypothesis has to be considered. This is that there is a group of patients without psychosis who have their pain as a result of thought processes. These patients could be said to have hallucinations of pain, since there is no external cause; or they can be regarded as having pain as a conversion symptom. The latter notion of pain as a hysterical symptom dates back for centuries and was described, for example, by Sydenham (41). Freud (9) accounted for pain as a conversion symptom and there are some patients who actually describe the genesis of pain as an idea in such a way that tension theories seem to be at least improbable. The obvious inference is that the pain resulted from that idea. Freud (9), for example, related how a man watched his brother having his ankylosed hip straightened under anesthetic. At the moment that the joint was freed a loud crack was heard and the observer felt the pain down the side of his own leg. Beck (3), quite incidentally, describes several comparable instances in his writing on cognitive therapy. I have also described (21) such a case and occasionally encountered others. We do not have to argue that pains due to thoughts are necessarily hysterical but, at least, we must recognize the category of pains due to thought processes and not having the characteristics of psychotic hallucinations. In practice it seems likely that these pains are most often hysterical in origin, serving a conversion function, but no sufficient analysis has been done as yet.

Further evidence in favor of the notion that many pains are hysterical in origin comes from three sources. First, it has long been known that, in some primitive societies, men take to bed when their wives are due to give birth and utter cries of pain (32). This is known as the couvade. A more sophisticated version of pain during a wife's pregnancy is noted in the form of toothache in English miners (7, 4) and abdominal pain in East Indian soldiers (2) and Australian and English men (43, 44), as well as various pains in Americans (5). Such pains require the notion of pain due to an idea.

Secondly, there is a link between patients with conversion symptoms and subsequent pain. Rawnsley and Loudon (31) described the medical state of a number of islanders from Tristan da Cunha who were evacuated to Britain when their island was threatened with a volcanic eruption. In 1938-1939 a Norwegian expedition had visited the island and found many of the inhabitants were having hysterical spells or attacks. The names of the afflicted were recorded. Twenty-five years later in Britain, Rawnsley and Louden found that a number of patients complained particularly of headaches and other pains. They were in many cases, and significantly often, the same people as those who had the hysterical spells. The same link between conversion symptoms and pain appears in many patients who have profuse somatic and bodily complaints and are often described by internists and general physicians as polysymptomatic. Some of these patients overlap with pain clinic patients. Guze and his colleagues (11, 51) have systematically described the extreme form of this pattern and called it Briquet's syndrome, after a nineteenth century physician prominent in the study of hysteria. The criteria of Guze required the patient to have at least thirty-five symptoms arising before the age of 25 from some nine different symptom areas. There are altogether ten available symptom areas listed. One of these symptom areas or groups includes classical motor conversion symptoms. Five of the groups include pain in one part or another.

It appears valid and necessary to think of pain as at times a hysterical conversion symptom. It will not often be directly accounted for in each individual case by a clear sequence of thoughts producing it. Moreover it is frequently unwise to take this view of the patient's pain precipitately. But treatment of chronic pain which fails to recognize this possibility will be doomed to produce many bad consequences, including excessive operations, unwise prescribing, inappropriate behavior therapy, and medical frustration.

EFFECTS OF PAIN

The discussion of pain so far has centered upon psychological causes of pain. Before reviewing the available treatment, it is important to draw the picture of the other side of the coin. Chronic pain from defined physical lesions is frequently debilitating. Mitchell (25) noted this in the following description of a man who had suffered a nerve lesion.

> He begged at times to be killed, at others to go home.... Sometimes he would lie open-eyed, regarding furiously the passers-by who shook his bed as they walked, every movement seeming to add to his torment... (later).... Under active treatment the pain lessened, but... From being a man of gay and kindly temper, known in his company as a good natured jester, he became morose and melancholy, and complained that reading gave him vertigo, and that his memory of recent events was bad.

Others have recognized the same pattern. Patients with severe pain for appropriate physical reasons become anxious and depressed. However this point has been relatively neglected in the psychiatric literature. Nevertheless some reports do exist which testify to its importance. Swerdlow (40), from the pain clinic in Salford, England, noted that persistent pain, as from postherpetic neuralgia, produced psychological changes which were very hard to reverse. Woodforde and Merskey (50) found that psychiatric patients with lesions and pain were, in general, as anxious and depressed as psychiatric patients with pain but without lesions, while on some scales, for example obsessionality, the patients with lesions tended to be more depressed than those who only had a psychiatric complaint. Sternbach et al. (37) found similar patterns of equivalent neuroticism in patients with and without organic lesions which might have contributed to their low back pain. Sternbach and Timmermans (38) subsequently noted reduction of some scores on the MMPI in those patients who had had successful treatment.

It is not surprising that pain causes emotional changes when it is due to a physical lesion. We normally think of pain as being intended to promote rest and healing, but it has another biological function as well. In experiements with rats (27), if an electric current is put across bars of the floor of the cage the rats may turn around and bite each other. Aggression is one of the main responses to trauma that may cause pain. The evidence on this is reviewed by Ulrich (46, 47). Aggression in response to pain can be thought of as part of the "fight or flight" mechanism. It has an obvious biological purpose. I suspect that superficial pain will be more likely to give rise to aggression, while deep pain will be more likely to lead to rest. Whatever the exact position, it is important to recognize that pain is likely to cause emotional changes.

MANAGEMENT OF CHRONIC PAIN: INVESTIGATION

The first essential in management is to make as accurate a diagnosis as possible. This is obvious but sometimes neglected. A neurologist with skill and interest in clinical testing for sensory disturbances is an invaluable member of the tearm. Case history taking devoted to careful analysis of the history of the pain is also of fundamental importance. It does not take long to obtain a detailed history of the location of each pain or pains and also of its relation to food, exercise, sleep, medication, and emotional states and its subjective characteristics. This needs to be done in addition to the usual physical and psychiatric inquiries. I can think off-hand of several patients in whom careful neurological examination or a special knowledge of pain syndromes produced a specific diagnosis and assessment and radically affected the approach to the patient's management, which previously had been muddled and unsatisfactory.

Diagnosis here also includes assessment or evaluation of the quantitative significance of a lesion. This is a helpful guide to the relative importance of emotional and psychological factors.

The second essential in management is to accept the reality of the patient's pain. There are only a few cases in which the physician will be deceived by simulators if he does this, unless his practice is largely related to compensation claims. In the latter instance, even if doubts are entertained, perfect courtesy in examination and management is still necessary. Some reasons for not denying the validity of the patient's experience have already been considered. In addition, the careful inquiry which treats the patient's pain as pain and not as "imaginary" is always appreciated by the patient and establishes the lack of prejudice of the physician. Psychiatrists and psychologists are perhaps most often faced with patients who feel that the reality of their pain has been denied. A careful review of the pain and its pattern is almost always helpful in showing that the examiner is interested in the patient's experience and impartially concerned to help the individual with his problem or problems.

It is best to review both the physical and psychiatric history and examination on the basis of these general principles. Those who have the relevant skills may repeat part or all these inquiries or extend them. There should never be any hesitation in doing this or in calling for an additional relevant opinion if in doubt. In the psychiatric history it is important always to obtain an account from an additional person, such as a close relative, relating particularly to the way in which pain affects the patient's behavior and to his or her usual emotional characteristics and history and to the existence of any important emotional problems. Most cases of chronic pain, even those with quite a lengthy history, can be adequately reviewed to this extent in a period of 2 hr. Many are reasonably complete in less time. The review can be adjourned until some future time if necessary. When the review is complete the patient should be offered a provisional opinion in advance of further investigations, except only those involving the minimum risk such as venipuncture or plain x-rays. The opinion should include any specific diagnosis reached, e.g., postherpetic neuralgia, tension headache, or depression, in terms the patient can understand and without alarming him. It should be accompanied by an estimate of the relationship of the diagnosis to the patient's pain. If it is not possible to reach a reasonable provisional diagnosis immediately it is advisable to tell the patient. If I have not found evidence of psychiatric illness and there is also no evidence of physical illness I explain this to the patient, adding that I believe further observation is warranted. This can include psychological exploration by a series of interviews, regular mild analgesic treatment, or a trial of antidepressants, depending on the extent to which one or another of these approaches are indicated.

Chronic pain patients are underinvestigated in terms of history taking, even though their charts are thick, and overinvestigated and overtreated in terms of surgery, narcotics or other potent medication. It is important to avoid these errors, but of course clear indications for more extensive investigation should be taken up promptly and fully, and after that the matter of investigation should be put on one side and not repeated unless the symptoms change or they do not respond as anticipated to the treatments judged appropriate. In that case, after due trial, the diagnosis must be reviewed.

Many centers and practictioners find it advantageous to arrange "a complete pain workup," perhaps as an inpatient, and certainly to solicit several types of specialist opinion. Besides the approach outlined, this may include formal psychological testing and intravenous barbituate pain testing (49). The first of these, e.g., with the MMPI, can be helpful in confirming clinical formulations and is a valuable and harmless research tool in the comparative analysis of patient groups. The second is a way of demonstrating that patients with regional pain of psychological origin may still have persisting skin tenderness at the first level of anesthesia (eyelash areflexia), while deep tenderness, which is physically based, persists into more profound anesthesia. I have only seen intravenous barbituate testing on two occasions, but it deserves further clinical attention and there is a need for more reports on it.

SPECIFIC SITUATIONS

The approach to management which has so far been outlined constitutes a basis for treatment and serves as part of the treatment. Insecurity, resentment, or despair, which can all be found in patients with pain, are ameliorated by the acceptance and understanding which are provided by careful sympathetic investigation and discussion. A positive transference, or at least a less negative one, is established and serves as the basis for further treatment. It is important not to promise too much or the positive transference can rebound embarrassingly and with justification upon the therapist, but equally it is desirable to have established a relationship of professional care and personal interest.

A few patients are accessible to highly specific treatments. The easiest is the use of antidepressants for those patients who have significant depression of the endogenous/psychotic type. Endogenous depression may be precipitated by external events like bereavement, but tends to have its own momentum and responds well, usually, to medication and, if necessary, ECT. Specialist help is not essential for the management of endogenous depression provided suicide can be ruled out, but it should be readily obtained if required. The earlier discussion should have made it clear, however, that this is not a common cause of pain complaints.

Significant depression with pain is more often due to environmental stresses and personal interactions which produce the pattern of exogenous/neurotic depression. The latter can also benefit from antidepressants but less markedly then does endogenous depression. Attention should be given to personal conflicts, and an exploration conducted with relatives of sources of dispute and emotional difficulties. It is reasonable to undertake environmental manipulations if they are feasible or acceptable, but it is unwise to push these on the patient. Vigorous advice to change a job or spouse should not be given, but joint exploration of the problems with one another is de rigeur. The patient or client can then take the decision whether to keep the pain or status quo.

Anxiety causing pain generally follows the same rules of treatment as endogenous depression. Even antidepressants may be helpful (but not ECT) and, incidentally, anxiety and depression are nearly always found together in varying proportions. Few anxious patients are not depressed and few depressed patients are not anxious.

As was indicated earlier, anxiety and depression are sometimes due to pain of physical origin. Appropriate physical measures should then be pursued, ranging from cutaneous counterstimulation to nerve blocks. Non-narcotic analgesics should be given on a regular round-the-clock basis rather than occasionally and some phenothiazines are helpful in the management of such patients (24, 42). The phenothiazines have an analgesic action that should only be used for chronic pain which has failed to respond to milder measures. They are not useful for the treatment of emotional states associated with pain. Their best use is as a sedative analgesic at night which gives the patient the opportunity to sleep better and to be less worn down by pain during the day. They have some tendency to cause depression and therefore it is always advisable to combine them with a modest dose of an antidepressant as well. Care has to be taken to avoid the cumulative anticholinergic side effects of these two types of drugs.

Antidepressants can also be given an empirical trial even without phenothiazines. On the whole they cause less trouble than surgery and it is particularly desirable to avoid polysurgery in patients with chronic pain.

With hypochondriacal and demanding patients, of whom there are many in pain clinics, and where the diagnosis is fundamentally one of hysteria, or if the term is preferred, "abnormal illness behavior," the utmost restraint has to be practiced with regard to all physical procedures, especially surgery. Although surgeons must be the best judges of whom they should operate upon, a strong case exists for the view that no pain surgery should be attempted on patients who have not had a complete psychiatric assessment and study with psychological testing. The benefits of any medical treatment, including psychotherapy, are likely to be small. The best policy is to adopt an attitude of support, simple counseling and guidance with the use of nontraumatic methods of treatment. Placebos should not be despised and acupuncture need not be rejected (although it has better uses), but the yield from all treatments is poor. Nevertheless benefit to the patient is substantial if damaging procedures are avoided.

Perhaps the most difficult problem of all has to do with the patients who have repeated surgery for a single painful area. Originally, 20 years and as many operations ago, there may have been a justifiable reason for surgery. Thereafter continuation of pain leads to successive operations, which leave the patient no better, or only better for 2 to 3 months, or sometimes just 2 to 3 days, or even hours. Local signs of organic disease (impaired innervation, neuromata) are scanty, doubtful or absent. The patient is dependent or beseeching, not necessarily dramatic. The pain is continuous, severe, and sometimes eased by narcotics. It is hard to know whether the personality causes pain or vice versa. It is tempting to speculate that autonomous pain, based on irreversible activity in the spinal cord or central nervous system, has been established; or else the syndrome is hysterical. The only sure conclusion is that further surgery will temporarily appease the patient but not allay the pain. It is easy to be wise after the event—especially when the event is the last of twenty. Supportive management, and when possible the withdrawal of narcotics, are usually the only worthwhile possibilities and the patient should be discouraged from touring world famous centers for further opinions.

Patients like the above are not the only ones who develop narcotic addiction. Others with defined lesions may have been placed on opiates which have been long continued. In such cases the opiates can be withdrawn provided that active treatment with sedative phenothiazines and anti-depressants is instituted to cover the withdrawal phase. Benzodiazepines can be used simultaneously, although they should not be prescribed indefinitely, and indeed there are some pain patients fuddled from their chronic use in conjunction with codeine, barbiturates, and meprobamate, all of which should normally be gradually discontinued. Such measures normally require admission to a suitably interested pain clinic or psychiatric ward. In general, chronic pain not associated with terminal illness should not be treated with narcotics. I have seen a very small number of patients with chronic pain who did not raise their dose of codeine or opiates and maintained good function with the help of these drugs. But such cases are exceptionally few. If opiates are withdrawn the substitution of analgesic mixtures of the type described can often be helpful, provided it is done with suitable attention to the detail of side effects and that the patients, thereby, become much less confused.

I have seen only four patients among many with chronic pain in whom it seemed that the withdrawal of narcotics left them worse overall than before.

The pain of terminal illness requires brief mention only, not because it is unimportant but because the basic principles are mostly similar to those already outlined. Recent reports have described the approach which has been found helpful (12, 33). First, perhaps the most important special point is to enable the patient to ventilate his or her feelings and anxieties to a caring physician who is prepared to be open with the individual. Secondly, the use of opiates need not be avoided and should, if necessary, be liberal. Nevertheless it is useful to use an antidepressant or phenothiazines also.

GENERAL MEASURES

Certain psychiatric treatments may be specific or general in their effects, perhaps because they entail the engendering of confidence and some placebo response as well as precise influences upon particular problems. Psychotherapy falls into such a category. It may be precise if it deals with specific complaints and emotional difficulties, or general if it provides an atmosphere of interest and support. There is such a wide range of psychotherapy, from individual types of treatment to group approaches, that no brief account could be adequate. The salient points of reference are: first, dealing with current conflicts and patterns of life adjustments by individual psychotherapy can be worthwhile; secondly, supportive approaches are more often all that can be usefully employed; and thirdly, group treatment has been praised but not yet shown to be very successful (30). Perhaps that is because the latter has been used for relatively difficult problems and with due appreciation that such patients could not be radically altered. Patients with chronic pain and depression show evidence of marital maladjustment (20, 26) and family therapy is relevant in such cases and beginning to be tried (16). Cognitive therapy (3, 16) is one version of psychotherapy, also not much used yet for pain, and deserves to be further investigated. Behavior therapy has been reported on (8), but its successes are very limited in the type of patients for whom it has so far been thought appropriate. It entails, moreover, a fundamental neglect of the patient's experience, which is simply likely to lead to the patient, who is not captive, discontinuing treatment without benefit. General rehabilitative measures are to be preferred. Lastly, biofeedback has been employed in a number of pain syndromes. There are numerous reports that it helps migraine and tension headaches. The best controlled study of the former known to me (15) concluded that the benefits were no better than with placebo. But it is a benign treatment and requires further exploration with such syndromes as backache.

CONCLUSIONS

The importance of the emotions in increasing chronic pain ought not to be in doubt in view of the extensive evidence on the matter. Nor should the importance be questioned of pain of physical origin in producing depression. The relevant psychiatric treatments span the range of psychiatric procedures and have to be selected according to their particular applicability in each case. A minority of patients can benefit substantially. There is, lastly, an important group of patients with chronic pain for whom the most useful approach is based on careful sympathetic assessment, supportive relationships, and very conservative therapy.

REFERENCES

1. Banks, M.H., Beresford, S.H.A., Morrell, D.C., Waller, J.J., and Watkins, C.J. Factors influencing demand for primary medical care in women aged 20-40 years; a preliminary report. *Int. J. Epidemiol.* 4, 189-195 (1975).

2. Bardhan, P.N. The fathering syndrome. *Armed Forces Med. J.* 20 (1965); The couvade syndrome. *Br. J. Psychol.* 111, 908-909 (1965).
3. Beck, A.T. *Cognitive Therapy and the Emotional Disorders.* International Univer. Press, New York, 1976.
4. Crann, P. personal communication, 1965.
5. Curtis, J.L. A psychiatric study of 55 expectant fathers. *U.S. Armed Forces Med. J.* 6, 937-950 (1955).
6. Delaplaine, R., Ifabumuyi, O.I., Merskey, H., and Zarfas, J. Significance of pain in psychiatric hospital patients, *Pain* 4, 361-366 (1978).
7. Dennis, N., Henriques, F., and Slaughter, C. *Coal is our Life.* Eyre and Spottiswoode, London, 1956.
8. Fordyce, W.E. Pain viewed as learned behaviour, in *Advances in Neurology,* vol. 4, J.J. Bonica, ed. Raven Press, New York, 1974, pp. 415-423.
9. Freud, S. Studies in hysteria, in *Complete Psychological Works. 1893-1895.* (standard ed.), vol. 2. Hogarth Press, London, 1955.
10. Gomez, J. and Dally, P. Psychologically mediated abdominal pain in surgical and medical outpatient clinics. *Br. Med. J.* 1, 1451-1453 (1977).
11. Guze, S.B. The role of follow-up studies: Their contribution to diagnostic classification as applied to hysteria. *Semin. Psychiatry* 2, 392-402 (1970).
12. Hackett, T.P. and Weisman, A.D. The treatment of the dying. *Curr. Psychiatr. Ther.* 2, 121-126 (1962).
13. Hanvik, J.L. MMPI profiles in patients with low-back pain, in *Basic Readings on the MMPI in Psychology and Medicine.* G.S. Welsh and W.G. Dahlstrom, eds. Oxford Univ. Press, London, 1956, pp. 499-504.
14. Jamison, K., Ferrer-Brechner, M.T., Brechner, V.L., and McCreary, C.P. Correlation of personality profile with pain syndrome, in *Advances in Pain Research and Therapy,* vol 1. Raven Press, New York, 1976, pp. 317-321.
15. Jessup, B.A. Autogenic relaxation and hand-temperature biofeedback for migraine. Ph.D. Thesis, Univ. of Western Ontario, 1978.
16. Khatami, M. and Rush, A.J. A pilot study of the treatment of out-patients with chronic pain: Symptom control, stimulus control, and social system intervention, *Pain,* 5, 163-172 (1978).
17. Klee, G.D., Ozelis, S., Greenberg, I., and Gallant, L.J. Pain and other somatic complaints in a psychiatric clinic. *Md. State Med. J.* 8, 188-191 (1959).
18. McEwan, B.W., DeWilde, F.W., Dwyer, B., Woodforde, J.M., Bleasel, K., and Connelly, T.J. The pain clinic: A clinic for the management of intractable pain. *Med. J. Aust.* 52, 676-682 (1965).
19. Merskey, H. The characteristics of persistent pain in psychological illness. *J. Psychosom. Res.* 9, 291-298 (1965).
20. Merskey, H. Psychiatric patients with persistent pain. *J. Psychosom. Res.* 9, 299-309 (1965).
21. Merskey, H. Psychological aspects of pain. *Postgrad. Med. J.* 44 (1968).
22. Merskey, H. Psychological aspects of pain relief; hypotherapy; psychotropic drugs, in *Relief of Intractable Pain,* 2nd ed. M. Swerdlow, ed. Excerpta Medica, Amsterdam (1978).
23. Merskey, H. and Boyd, D.B. Emotional adjustment and chronic pain. *Pain,* 5, 173-178 (1978).
24. Merskey, H. and Hester, R.N. The treatment of chronic pain with psychotropic drugs. *Postgrad. Med. J.* 594-598 (1972).
25. Mitchell, S.W. *Injuries of Nerves and Their Consequences.* Dover, New York, 1965.
26. Mohamed, S.N., Weisz, G.M., and Waring, E.M. The relationship of chronic pain to depression, marital adjustment and family dynamics. *Pain* 5, 285-292 (1978).
27. O'Kelly, L.E. and Steckley, L.C. A note on long enduring emotional responses in the rat. *J. Psychol.* 8, 125 (1939); cited by Ulrich et al. (47).

28. Pilowsky, I., Chapman, C.R., and Bonica, J.J. Pain, depression and illness behaviour in a pain clinic population. *Pain* 4, 183-192 (1977).
29. Pilowsky, I. and Spence, N.D. Pain and illness behaviour: A comparative study. *J. Psychosom. Res.* 20, 131-134 (1976).
30. Pinsky, J.J. Psychodynamics and psychotherapy in the treatment of patients with chronic intractable pain, in *Pain: Research and Treatment.* B.L. Crue, ed. Academic Press, New York, 1975.
31. Rawnsley, K. and Loudon, J.B. Epidemiology of mental disorder in a closed community. *Br. J. Psychiatry* 110, 830-839 (1964).
32. Reik, T. *Ritual: Psychoanalytical Studies.* Hogarth Press, London, 1914.
33. Saunders, G. Terminal care, in *Medical Oncology,* K.D. Bagshawe, ed. Blackwells, Oxford, 1975.
34. Smith, D.P., Pilling, L.F., Pearson, J.S., Rushton, J.C., Goldstein, N.P., and Gibilisco, J.A. A psychiatric study of atypical facial pain. *Can. Med. Assoc. J.* 100, 286-291 (1969).
35. Spear, F.G. Pain in psychiatric patients. *J. Psychosom. Res.* 11, 187-193 (1967).
36. Sternbach, R.A. *Pain Patients: Traits and Treatment.* Academic Press, New York, 1974.
37. Sternbach, R.A., Murphy, R.W., Akeson, W.H., and Wolf, S.R. Chronic low back pain: The "low-back loser." *Postgrad. Med.* 53, 125-138 (1973).
38. Sternbach, R.A. and Timmermans, G. Personality changes associated with reduction of pain. *Pain* 1, 177-181 (1975).
39. Swanson, D.W., Floreen, A.C., and Swenson, W.M. Program for managing chronic pain. II. Short-term results. *Proc. Mayo Clin.* 51, 409-411 (1976).
40. Swerdlow, M. The pain clinic. *Br. J. Clin. Pract.* 9, 403-407 (1972).
41. Sydenham, T. Discourse concerning hysterical and hypochondriacal distempers, in *Dr. Sydenham's Complete Method of Curing Almost All Diseases, and Description of Their Symptoms. To which are now added Five Discourses of the Same Author Concerning the Pleurisy, Gout, Hysterical Passion, Dropsy, and Rheumatism,* 3rd. ed. Newman and Rich Parker, London, 1967, p. 149.
42. Taub, A. and Collins, W.F. Observations on the treatment of denervation dysethesia with psychotropic drugs: Postherpetic neuralgia, anaesthesia dolorosa, peripheral neuropathy, in *Advances in Neurology,* vol. 4. Raven Press, New York, 1974, pp. 309-315.
43. Trethowan, W.H. and Conlon, M.F. The couvade syndrome. *Br. J. Psychiatry* 111, 57-76 (1965).
44. Trethowan, W.H. The couvade syndrome—Some further observations. *J. Psychosom. Res.* 12, 107-115 (1968).
45. Twycross, R.G. Relief of terminal pain. *Br. Med. J.* 4, 212-214 (1975).
46. Ulrich, R.E. Pain as a cause of aggression. *Am. Zool.* 6, 643-662 (1966).
47. Ulrich, R.E., Hutchinson, P.R., and Azrin, N.H. Pain—Elicited aggression. *Psychol. Res.* 15, 111-126 (1965).
48. Van Boxtel, H. and Roozeveld VanderVen, J. Differential EMG activity in subjects with muscle contraction headaches related to mental effort. *Headache* 17, 233-237 (1978).
49. Walters, J.A. Psychiatric considerations of pain, in *Neurological Surgery.* J. Youmans, ed. W.B. Saunders, Philadelphia, 1973, ch. 86, pp. 1615-1645.
50. Woodforde, J.M. and Merskey, H. Personality traits of patients with chronic pain. *J. Psychosom. Res.* 16, 173-178 (1972).
51. Woodruff, R.A., Jr. Hysteria: An evaluation of objective diagnostic criteria by the study of women with chronic medical illnesses. *Br. J. Psychiatry* 114, 1115-1119 (1968).

CHAPTER 8

Personality and the Relief of Chronic Pain: Predicting Surgical Outcome

W. LYNN SMITH
DONALD L. DUERKSEN

Although chronic pain is perhaps the most widespread and least understood symptom on the health care delivery scene today, traditional medical and surgical procedures aimed at chronic pain relief have produced only limited success. There is a growing awareness among health care professionals that further advances will require a multidisciplinary approach with a long look given to personality contributing factors which influence outcome.

Neurosurgeon Norman Shealy (7) estimates that "60% of the chronic pain patients who are frequenting clinics across the country...represent failures of surgical intervention techniques for pain relief." According to Benjamin Crue (2), another neurosurgeon and expert in the study of pain, "Clinicians, especially surgeons,...might well approach chronic pain in most human syndromes, in the absence of malignant neoplasms, from the standpoint of possible ways to reprogram the 'central computer' rather than remaining fixed in the acute pain organic medical model."

Low back pain is one of the most frequently encountered chronic pain syndromes and success rates continue to be poor in spite of recent medical and surgical advances. As psychologist Richard Sternbach and his associates (8) have emphasized, the continuation of pain may be caused by a failure to recognize and treat low back pain as an illness with substantial psychological components.

Surgical procedures aimed at the relief of other pain syndromes, though less frequent and less studied, present similar problems in outcome.

In the Cortical Function Laboratory at Porter Memorial Hospital and Swedish Medical Center in Denver, our experience with patients suffering from chronic pain developed over the last few years as surgeons began referring patients who had failed to recover as expected from "technically successful" surgery. We were called upon initially to document the presence or absence of personality characteristics which may have interfered with the recovery from these procedures aimed at pain relief. However, the surgeons' growing awareness of the importance of personality factors contributing to the chronic pain syndrome soon led to a series of referrals, prior to surgery, for predictive statements regarding expected treatment outcome.

Prior to surgery, the patients were interviewed and given a neuropsychological test battery consisting of standard psychodiagnostic measures. Predictions for or against postoperative pain alleviation were made prior to surgery and these predictions were based on the objective test results, as well as our subjective clinical judgments from prior experience with patients suffering from chronic pain. Six months following surgery, the surgeons rated each patient according to success or failure of pain alleviation. This assessment was based on a complete medical evaluation and included the patients' own subjective reports, as well as objective information including reduced need for pain medication and increased activity level.

After we had accumulated results on the first twenty-three surgical patients for whom we had made predictions, we initiated the present study in order to explore further the relationship between certain personality variables in chronic pain patients and to develop a valid psychometric index for the prediction of success or failure of surgical intervention aimed at the relief of chronic pain.

Of the first twenty-three patients who had undergone surgery for the relief of pain, the postsurgical course of twenty-one had been accurately predicted, an encouraging result that led us to a detailed re-analysis of the test protocols of the surgical patients. It should be noted that, as a consequence of predictions of surgical nonsuccess, some physicians chose to postpone indefinitely any surgical intervention, thus restricting the possibility of verifying our predictions regarding those patients. Also, four patients had to be dropped from the study due to the intervening variable of physical complications. For example, one young man who appeared well on the road to recovery, fell off a skate board and reinjured his back.

From the remaining nineteen patient protocols, a preliminary Pain Assessment Index was developed, which was used along with our clinical predictions, and was continually refined as patients were added to the initial sample group.

DEVELOPMENT OF THE PAIN ASSESSMENT INDEX

A brief review of the research involving the use of psychological tests for predicting response to procedures aimed at pain relief showed that while the results have been somewhat inconsistent and occasionally contradictory, a few factors have consistently shown predictive significance, correlating well with our initial data.

Wiltse and Roccio (10) found the elevated Hy and Hs scales on the MMPI to be the best psychometric predictors of non-postsurgical relief. Wiffling et al. (9) reported similar findings and suggested that patients with less neurotic symptomatology recovered more quickly. Hanvik (4) had earlier identified the "conversion V" MMPI profile, formed by an elevated Hs and Hy with a relatively lower D scale score, which characterized cases of presumed backache of psychological origin and also noted a slight rise on the Pt scale. Working with cases of low back pain, Blumetti and Modesti (1) also noted the predictive value of the Hs and Hy scales of the MMPI, as well as the Form and Symbiosis scores from the Rorschach. Using Fisher and Cleveland's (3) Barrier score from the Rorschach, they found it to be significantly lower in the unimproved group. They found no significant differences between the groups on the descriptive variables of age, sex, socioeconomic status, IQ, length of symptomatology, or type of surgery performed.

In addition to the factors suggested by the previous research, a variety of other variables were checked for their predictive value. Leary (5), in adapting the MMPI to his own system of interpersonal diagnosis, used several combinations of MMPI scales, two of which appeared likely candidates for tapping the personality dimensions involving the perception of pain. A Ma minus D score was suggested to indicate strength and confidence versus weakness and immobilization. We adapted this difference score and used a D–Ma + 50, to change the direction and raise the scores to a level comparable with the "T" score range of single clinical scales. Leary also suggested that the Hs–Pt score brought forward an indication of the balance between concerns over physical health versus concerns over emotional problems, and felt that relatively higher scores were obtained by psychosomatic patients. In line with the other difference score, we used Hs–Pt + 50. We also checked the predictability of each of these scales on a single basis.

We felt that the Rorschach, as a valuable clinical technique, might show factors of predictive significance in addition to the Barrier scores mentioned by Blumetti and Modesti (1). We were interested largely in easily recognizable Rorschach features rather than detailed factors involving extended scoring, as this would diminish the usefulness of the index as a screening device. Rorschach content was checked in three groups. Anatomy responses have been considered a sign of somatic conern and were the category we felt had the most promise. Content suggesting passive/dependent traits, such as diminuative animals, cute figures, people perceived dancing or kissing, etc., were classed under Hys. responses. Human content in general was also checked to see if the assumed self-absorption of pain patients had affected the extent of Human perception on the Rorschach. Card "shock," the relative difficulty in forming a percept and/or the inability to produce an adequate response is a feature often noted in Rorschach records of generally neurotic style, and this feature was checked for shock to Cards II, III, VII, and IX. A detailed discussion of these features has been presented by Phillips and Smith (6).

The Street Gestalt Completion Test, in the absence of organic conditions, gives a roughly accurate indication of the relative dominance of analytical versus intuitive thought processes, the latter of which is commonly thought dominant in hysterical individuals, and this score was checked as well.

In addition, the descriptive variables of age, sex, type of surgery, and inpatient versus outpatient status were examined.

Our final patient sample of 31 included 23 females, whose ages ranged from 24 to 66 with a mean of 41.7, and 8 males, age 26 to 65 with a mean of 43.1. All but one were Caucasian and all were members of the middle socioeconomic class. All patients had been suffering from chronic pain and all underwent surgery as follows: for low-back pain: 17, for neck pain: 1, for Thoracic Outlet Syndrome: 6, open-heart surgery: 2, hand surgery: 3, abdominal surgery: 1, sinus surgery: 1.

It is important to note that all but three patients were facing their first surgery directed at the relief of chronic pain. Only the hand surgeries had one or more similar surgeries in the past.

As described earlier, all patients had been administered a neurophsycological test battery and clinical predictions had been made prior to surgery regarding the postsurgical course. These predictions were made known to the surgeon, but not to the patient. The success or failure of pain alleviation was rated by the surgeon, using the subjective and objective criteria mentioned earlier, after at least a 6 month recovery period.

A total of 24 variables or combinations of variables were analyzed for their predictive capabilities. A Chi Square test of significance was performed for each variable, as well as a Point-Biserial Correlation Coefficient. The six significant factors which emerged, all from the MMPI, are presented in Table 1 with their correlation coefficients. The cut-off score, significance level, number of false positives and negatives, and percentage of correct prediction for each scale is presented in Table 2.

As expected, and consistent with previous findings, our results showed elevations on both the Hy and Hs scales of the MMPI to be highly significant. The presence of the classical "conversion V" configurations was not found to be significant; however, any configuration in which the Hs scale was equal to

Table 1. Point-Biserial Correlation Coefficients of the Significant MMPI Variables and the Final Index Score versus Outcome

Variable	Correlation
Hs scale	0.731
Hy scale	0.570
D scale	0.594
Hs–Hy + 50	0.413
Hs–Pt + 50	0.418
D–Ma + 50	0.499
Index	0.834

Table 2. Chi Square Significance Level, Cutoff Score, and Predictive Efficiency in Terms of False Positives and Negatives, and Percent Correctly Identified for each Variable

Variable	Significance (P≤)	Cutoff	False Positives	False Negatives	% Correct
Hs scale	0.001	(grouped)	-	-	-
		≥70T	5	0	83.9
Hy scale	0.005	≥70T	10	0	67.7
	0.006	≥75T	3	4	77.4
D scale	0.0003	≥60T	3	2	83.9
Hs–Hy + 50	0.003	≥50	6	2	74.2
Hs–Pt + 50	0.002	≥61	5	2	77.4
D–Ma + 50	0.01	≥56	5	3	74.2
Clinical predictions	-	-	3	0	90.3
Index	0.00001	≥13	0	2	93.5

or greater than the Hy scale (Hs–Hy + 50≥50) was significant. Somewhat unexpected was the high significance of the D scale. Both the D–Ma and the Hs–Pt scores proved to be significant.

Although showing a directional trend, the Street Gestalt Completion test did not show high significance. The descriptive variables of age, sex, type of surgery, and in- or outpatient status at the time of testing also proved to be nonsignificant. None of the factors taken from the Rorschach showed predictive significance, although, again, some directional trends were noted.

Using the six significant factors in Table 1, the Pain Assessment Index was constructed as follows. Linear regression equations and data inspection were used to establish cutoff points for five of the factors. The Hs scale was used on a continuous basis because of its high correlation. Index points were assigned as follows: 1 point for each 5T that the Hs scale exceeded 55T and –1 point for each 5T that the Hs scale was below 55T; 7 points if the Hy scale exceeded 75T or 2 points if the Hy scale was 71–75T; 3 points if the D scale exceeded 60T; 2 points if the Hs scale was greater than or equal to the Hy scale; 2 points if the D–Ma + 50 was greater than 55; and 2 points if the Hs–Pt + 50 was greater than 60. Multiple linear regression equations and data inspection were used to establish the weighting points for each factor.

On our sample of 31, this index produces scores ranging from 0 to 21 with a mean of 9.6. The postsurgically improved group produced scores from 0 to 12 with a mean of 5.5 and the unimproved group ranged from 10 to 21 with a mean of 17.1. Using a cutoff of 13 or above for a poor prognosis, the index correctly identified 29 of the 31 cases, with 2 false negatives and no false positives, and produced a Chi Square significance of $p < 0.00001$ and a Point-Biserial Correlation Coefficient of $r_{pbi} = 0.834$. These results are produced in Tables 1 and 2 for comparison with the individual factors.

It is interesting to note that our original clinical predictions erred in the direction of false positives, predicting continued pain for three patients who actually achieved significant pain reduction following surgery, whereas the Pain Index is a bit more lenient erring in the direction of false negatives, predicting a successful postsurgical result for two patients who did, in fact, show no significant pain reduction.

One additional point of importance concerning the nature of our patient sample should be presented. All patients had been experiencing chronic pain and all had demonstrable physical problems for which surgical intervention was planned. However, as most of these individuals were facing their first surgery aimed at chronic pain relief, they are not a representative sample of the type of chronic pain patients being seen in pain clinics across the country. It is our impression that the individuals we have identified as showing a poor prognosis for pain alleviation are the ones most likely to fit the pattern of the typical chronic benign pain patient.

Although our sample group is relatively small, the similarity of our findings with the previous research and the consistent significance of the additional factors we examined enables us to sketch a preliminary if somewhat speculative picture of the chronic pain patient for whom surgery will bring little or no relief.

One of the most outstanding features noted is the extent to which these individuals have focused their worries and fears onto their bodies as opposed to those whose anxiety and/or depression is primarily bound up with their thoughts and subjective experiences. The other remarkable feature is the distinct passive/dependent makeup of these patients. It appears that at least one of these factors must be present in the personality of the patient before a continuing chronic pain syndrome is possible from a psycho-emotional standpoint. In addition, depression appears to play a highly significant role, although conscious representations may be very slight. There seems to be very little flexibility in these individuals' defenses against anxiety, that is, they appear forced to remain locked into one defensive posture.

In short, these individuals appear passive, helpless, depressed, and seem to see themselves as victims of their own bodies rather than masters of them. This constellation of factors, we believe, represents an inability for self-mobilization. In other words, the individual's passive nature leads him to rely on external techniques to change his internal perceptions, or put at another level, the depressed person attributes to external events internal feelings of being torn, worn, and full of despair, his unconscious hope is that the internal state can be altered by body change. Mood and body image are inextricably bound in the "depressive equivalent." This dynamic view offers a strong case for psychotherapy as a basic treatment approach for the chronic benign pain patient.

In most cases, it seems that pain has, or has had at one time, a physical basis. As Benjamin Crue (2) has stated, "chronic benign pain is a perception, not a sensation," and when the original physical source is removed, the experience of pain often continues. It is important to note that in these individuals, the "pain" is real, they are not malingerers, although unconscious secondary gain, such as the fulfillment of dependency needs, does often occur. It is also important to point out that although these individuals do not present a picture of "psychological health," neither are they the epitome of "psychological illness." Others may simply have their anxiety organized in a different fashion.

If this brief picture is correct, it raises serious questions regarding surgical intervention for chronic pain relief in the absence of thorough neuropsychological screening. Our findings suggest that there is a direct relationship between the neuropsychological indices of the patient's capacity for self-mobilization and the subsequent treatment outcome.

An alternative to repetitive and frequently unsuccessful surgical interventions for chronic pain is being offered by innovative pain control centers and clinics in which interdisciplinary methods of treatment require much more self-mobilization from the patient than do the more passive and less personal techniques, such as transcutaneous electrical nerve stimulators, acupuncture, pain cocktails, and surgery. Many patients need to become committed to and involved with their treatment in order to manage their anxiety and break themselves free of the hold that chronic pain has on them.

Continued investigation of both personality variables and life situations is needed to correlate their influences on medical and surgical efforts aimed at chronic pain relief. Also needed is a study of those patients not regarded by their physicians as posing problems as to surgical outcome, to insure that future assessment procedures will advance to the point of not only reliably predicting surgical outcome, but also provide health care professionals with specific suggestions as to success enhancing, self-mobilizing techniques. Further, neuropsychological assessment indices of the future may prove useful even in suggesting alternative nonsurgical procedures for pain reduction.

REFERENCES

1. Blumetti, A.E. and Modesti, M.M. Psychological predictors of success or failure of surgical intervention for intractable back pain, in *Advances in Pain Research and Therapy*, J. Bonica and D. Able-Fessard, eds. Raven Press, New York, 1975.
2. Crue, B., Jr. The continuing crisis in pain research, in *Pain: Meaning and Management*, W. Lynn Smith, H. Merskey, and S.C. Gross, eds. Spectrum, New York, 1979.
3. Fisher, S. and Cleveland, S.E. *Body Image and Personality*. Van Nostrand Reinhold, New York, 1958.
4. Hanvik, L.H. MMPI profiles in patients with low-back pain. *J. Consulting Psychol.* 15, 350-353 (1951).
5. Leary, T. *Interpersonal Diagnosis of Personality*. Ronald Press, New York, 1957.
6. Phillips, L. and Smith, J.G. *Rorschach Interpretation: Advanced Technique*. Grune & Stratton, New York, 1953.
7. Shealy, C.N. *Pain Game*. Celestial Arts, Millrae, Calif., 1976.
8. Sternbach, R.A., Wolf, S.R., Murphy, R.W. and Akeson, W.H. Aspects of chronic low-back pain. *Psychosomatics* 14, 52-56 (1973).
9. Wiffling, F.J., Klonoff, H., and Kofan, P. Psychological, demographic and orthopaedic factors associated with prediction of outcome of spinal fusion. *Clin. Orthopaed.* 90, 153-160 (1973).
10. Wiltse, L.L. and Roccio, P.D. Preoperative psychological tests as predictors of success of chemonucleolisis in the treatment of low-back syndrome. *J. Bone Joint Surg.* 57-A1, 478-483 (1975).

CHAPTER 9

Child Pain: Treatment Approaches

STEVEN C. GROSS
G. GALE GARDNER

INTRODUCTION

There is a notable lack of medical, nursing, and psychological literature on the subject of pain in children. Pediatric medical and nursing research deals almost exclusively with specific disease conditions, merely addressing pain symptomatically. For the most part, psychiatric and psychological investigations on the subject of pediatric pain narrowly fixate on the psychogenic mechanisms used by the child to meet dependency needs or to avoid attending school. A thorough search of medical literature dating from January 1970 to August 1975 produced 1380 articles on pain, while only 33 dealt with the subject of pediatric pain (12).

The current paper will present a brief overview of some of the fundamental psychological issues involved in pediatric pain. To date many of the most relevant questions have yet to be addressed, let alone conclusively answered.

Pain Perception

The precise age at which pain is first perceived is *still unknown*. Some authors claim that infants do not react to a pain stimulus until a week after delivery and then make only mass responses until 1 month of age (25). However, most evidence suggests that some degree of pain awareness is present from birth.

The infant's perception of pain is, in part, determined by the degree of cortical development. Some researchers suggest that a baby with an undeveloped cortex and a deeply anesthetized patient may both lack the cortical activity necessary to feel pain (35). Although infants may be unable to localize or to specifically identify the source of the pain it is easily demonstrated that from their first injection in the delivery room, active, full term infants react to the stimulation of needle punctures by withdrawal of the affected part and by vigorous crying. Therefore, it is believed that the stimulus reaches the thalamus and is referred to higher centers. Although a neonate reacts to certain stimului by crying, the pain may be felt, but probably is not remembered. More complete cortical development and full awakening are considered necessary for normal consciousness and remembrance of pain.

Researchers have correlated the anatomic maturation of myelinization with the physiological development necessary for pain responses. Although myelinization is only partially completed at birth, the process proceeds rapidly from the second or third week of life (26). It is important to note that myelinization proceeds at different rates among infants. Therefore, the working hypothesis that the neonate does not perceive nor remember pain during the first weeks of life certainly needs further investigation.

Shirkey found that on the first day after birth a relatively large amount of electrical stimulation is needed to evoke a pain response, while by the third month only half of the initial stimulation is necessary. Poznanski (3) has noted that many anesthesiologists still do not use general anesthesia until the infant reaches about 3 months of age, basing their decision partially on the assumption of reduced pain threshholds in neonates and infants. Peiper justifiably criticizes surgeons who, believing that neonates and infants are completely insensitive to pain, perform lengthy operations without anesthesia and continue to do so, contrary to everyday experience and to scientific data (30).

INDIVIDUAL AND GROUP DIFFERENCES

It is not appropriate to talk about the pain experience of children in global terms. Developmental age, prior painful experiences, ability to communicate, family interactions, psychological defense mechanisms, and chronic versus acute conditions are but some of the important variables to be considered with pediatric pain.

Each developmental level has its unique considerations. During the first weeks of life, gross reflexive behavioral responses to pain are the dominant mode of expression. Gradually, during the second and third months, voluntary movements become more frequent. Muscular withdrawal and crying are the infants' primary means of communicating pain. Toddlers may nonverbally communicate pain by clenching their lips, rocking, rubbing, opening their eyes widely, and exhibiting agitated or aggressive physical behaviors, such as kicking, hitting, or biting (16).

The preschool aged child's beginning verbal abilities are still limited, particularly when localizing and describing pain symptoms. When communicating directly with the preschool aged child the diagnostician should keep in mind the child's age-specific and possibly idiosyncratic language of pain. Terms such as "discomfort" or even "pain" may be quite foreign, whereas "hurt," "ouchie," and "boo-boo" are more understandable. Although the child may be able to give the diagnostician some valuable information regarding his pain if the questions are phrased in the age-appropriate vernacular, parents who are keenly aware of behavioral or dispositional changes in their children continue to be extremely valuable informants.

The preschooler's cognitive functioning level is concrete and egocentric. Pain is often perceived as a punishment for some wrong doing or bad thought. Painful therapeutic treatments given by the physician, nurse, or parent may be interpreted by the child as deliberate, hostile, and punishing events. Anxiety and tears accompanying preventive or therapeutic procedures may, in part, be the result of remorse for some known or presumed indiscretion perceived by the child.

It is difficult for the young child to comprehend the true meanings of his pain and to relate it to realistic future outcomes. Assuring a preschool aged child that the pain will go away sometime in the future may not be fully understood nor believed, depending upon his needs for immediate gratification, history of previous painful experiences, and cognitive development.

The fear of bodily injury among school aged children is well documented. Children at this age tend to exaggerate even minor bruises and injuries. When severe pain is involved, anxiety and fear of bodily harm and even death can be a major preoccupation. For many children around the age of ten and eleven anxiety and fear regarding loss of control seems to be a major component of their concept of pain. Schultz asked children of this age group to complete the statement, "Pain is...." Frequently stated responses included: "...being afraid," "...something you have no control of," "...you think it will never end" (32).

Sex typing also has its influence. Boys, in general, tend to proudly report that they felt "brave" when they had pain and girls more often said they felt "nervous" or "afraid" (32).

By school age, the child's cognitive functions allow him to better understand the reasons for his pain, if it is explained in terms and concepts to which he can relate. The child also better understands that pain can be time-limited.

ADULT RESPONSES TO PEDIATRIC PAIN

Medical and nursing personnel often deal with pediatric pain differently than they do with adult pain. This difference may be partially due to faulty pain evaluation procedures and persisting myths regarding pediatric pain. As an example, Swafford and Allan bluntly suggest that "young pediatric patients seldom need medication for the relief of pain after general surgery, they tolerate discomfort well" (35). Contrary to this advice, recent research findings seem to suggest that pain thresholds increase with age; the younger the child, the more susceptible he is to pain (17).

It is well known that children tend to be ambulatory after surgery significantly sooner than adults. This observation is used to justify the child's seeming ability to suffer less. Eland and Anderson note that because a child is on his feet quicker than his adult counterpart does not mean that the pain is less severe. Physical activity has long been recognized as one coping technique children use to distract themselves from unpleasant stimuli (12).

Eland reported that a surprisingly large number of postsurgical children were never given any medication for pain relief during their entire hospitalization. Analgesic medications prescribed for children tended to be considerably less potent than those given to adults with the same physical problem (even when taking into account proportionately lower children's dosages). In those cases where equivalent pain medications were prescribed, nurses tended to dispense and/or to offer prn medications less frequently to children than to adults (11).

Medical and nursing staffs often operate under the false assumptions that, unless the children can accurately identify and label his discomfort, is it nonexistent or need not be treated. Also, the notion that children should be spared from the "dangerous" addicting side effects of pain relieving medications ignores the fact that acute pain following an operation is usually of fairly short duration, seldom long enough for addiction to occur. The long term effects of overwhelming acute pain may have much more serious psychological effects than the carefully monitored, appropriate prescription and dispensation of analgesic medication.

PSYCHOSOCIAL EFFECTS

Children with recurrent pain tend, as a group, to demonstrate character-istics such as hostility, dependency, anxiety, excitability, and other generally negative reactions more frequently than do pain-free children.

Recurrent pain complaints among children are widely thought to reflect difficulties in coping with conflict and stress situations (1). Common sources of emotional difficulties include: psychological illness in one or both parents; marital discord among the parents; parental preoccupation with illness; parental absence; school problems; difficulty in handling aggressive, hostile, or sexual feelings; and unsatisfactory parent-child relationships (13).

According to Friedman, the variables of sex, family size, ordinal position, and IQ do not differentiate children with psychogenic pain from those whose complaints reflect organic problems. Most children with recurrent pain syndromes range from five to sixteen years. The mean age for boys is ten and one-half years; for girls it is eleven and one-half years. These children frequently come from families in which the parents are also prone to pain (13). Oster noted that these families have a tendency toward a general proneness to pain rather than specific bodily localizations of pain (29).

An important, though often unexpressed concern among children is their ongoing independence/dependence struggle. While striving for independ-ence, children in pain are faced with a condition which is seemingly beyond their control and which seriously restricts their thoughts, activities, and feelings of independence. Children with severe pain may even be angry with themselves for being ill (32). These children may be school conscious and worry about poor grades or failing; they may be socially conscious and worry about peer opinion; they may feel they are a burden on their family; they may resent being deprived of certain activities and privileges; and they may feel responsible for their painful condition.

Helping the child to help himself control pain is the key intervention strategy required to enhance the chances for physiological and psychological independence.

SECONDARY GAINS

Secondary gain is often mentioned as an aspect of child pain, particularly as it relates to school-phobic children. Berger (6) listed four general family characteristics of school phobics who manifest somatic pain complaints. (1) Parents reflect an overprotective, infantilizing attitude toward the affected child; insisting that the symptoms are organically caused; allowing no household responsibilities during symptomatic periods; complying with the child's dietary and other whims; and generally treating the child as if he were developmentally or intellectually younger than in actuality. (2) The child's choice of symptoms coincides with the family's style of responding to stress with somatic complaints; mothers are often considered by their families and by themselves as physically or emotionally in need of help; the mother also often complains of vague somatic pains. (3) Distorted opinions of an irresponsible or insensitive father are often held by other family members, which often is not the case in reality. (4) The occurrence of recent changes in the family is typical, e.g., older siblings leaving the home and causing a partial empty-next syndrome.

While keeping these family situations in mind, we must avoid drawing the erroneous conclusion that once the secondary gain conditions are controlled, the pain is also necessarily controlled. Even in cases of psychogenic pain, secondary gains may only be incidental consequences related to coping mechanisms for the relief of pain symptoms.

DEFENSE MECHANISMS

Denial and regression are common defense mechanisms which children use to help cope with pain. Regression is often employed by adults as well as by children. For many, approximating an earlier, more dependent period in one's life when our well being was protected, our anxieties were soothed, and our confidence in the power and goodness of others remained unshaken, may be seen as an effective alternative to the present, very unpleasant, and helpless pain situation. Behaviors linked to these earlier, protected years, such as demands to be held or fed, infantile speech patterns, requests for help in toileting and dressing, and needs for continuous supervision and companionship, may help reduce anxieties related to the loneliness of pain and, therfore, the extreme pain perception. Nonpathological regressive symptoms may have the double benefit of both reducing anxieties related to the present time and place, and also in helping to mobilize others to aid in a lonely defense against overpowering pain.

RECURRENT PAIN SYNDROMES

Apley suggests that, in contrast to adults, the only common sites of pain which occur over a considerable time in children are in the abdomen, limbs, and head (2). Low-back pain, for example, is rare in children.

Abdominal pain is the most frequent, recurrent, somatic complaint of children. It is reported in as many as one of nine school aged children (2). Yet most of these recurrent abdominal pains do not seem to have an organic basis. Only for about 5% of the children with recurrent abdominal pain were organic origins found (4).

Apley noted certain resemblances between young patients with abdominal, limb, or head pain. A large majority have no major physical disease to which the main presenting symptoms can be attributed; emotional disturbances are very common and their manifestations strikingly similar; the families are also prone to similar pains and to nervous disorders (5). Although the pains nearly always predominate in one site, in more than one-third of the cases pains occur also in one or both of the other sites, either at the same or at different times. Pains at one site are sometimes unexplainably substituted for pains at another (4).

Since organic causes are found for relatively few cases of recurrent pain in children, the physician usually assures the young patient and the anxious parent that the symptoms are "nothing to worry about," and that the child will "grown out of the problem." However, a large proportion of children with recurrent abdominal pains do not outgrow their painful symptoms. In long term follow-up studies, approximately one-third continue to have abdominal symptoms ten to 20 years later. One-third develop other recurrent, "nervous," pain complaints, such as migraine, other types of headache, or low back pain. Only the remaining one-third are relatively symptom free (10). Interestingly, in this study, a large number of the children with persistent abdominal symptoms had an extended period in adolescence without symptoms; however, in the majority of cases, chronic pain symptoms resurfaced in later years.

Reassurance and symptomatic treatment may seemingly help the child at the time, and also help the family, but it does not necessarily alter the long term prognosis.

Are childhood organic disorders which present with pain missed through faulty initial evaluations and only years later correctly diagnosed? In general, the initial investigation seems to be satisfactory; however, the management of nonorganic abdominal pains may be somewhat less consistent (36).

In the case of psychogenic pain, it is not enough for the physician to rule out organic disease or to assume the presence of underlying emotional difficulties. It is important to establish the nature of contributing psychological problems and to develop a treatment plan which can be carried out either by the pediatrician or through referral to a psychotherapist. Likewise, in the case of organic pain, it is not enough to tell the child, parents, and others that one must just expect a certain amount of pain. Here, too, there must be a careful plan for pain control. Otherwise, many children—and some parents—will experience severe or repeated organic pain in the context of preexisting emotional difficulties. Then the two problems may combine to give a clinical picture in which it is very difficult to assess the pain and, hence, more difficult to treat.

Of course we see combinations of organic and psychogenic pain not only in children whose organic pain is understood—as in postsurgical pain—but also in children with a past history of organic pain who now complain of exacerbation of the extent or severity of the pain without any obvious physical explanation for the change. Again, rapid assessment and initiation of treatment are essential in order to minimize further complications and set the child, as soon as possible, back on a course which focuses on growth and mastery rather than on the debilitating effects of pain.

TREATING PAIN IN CHILDREN

Given the complexity of working with children in pain, the physician must either be skilled in psychological assessment and treatment or must work closely with pediatric psychologists and psychiatrists who are competent in these areas. Obviously the mental health professionals must recognize the bounds of their competence in the area of pain and must be able to consult with the pediatrician concerning medical aspects of the situation. Where two or more people are involved, the division of labor will vary, depending on the source of the pain and the nature and extent of related medical and psychological issues. Since problems of pain often involve frequent changes in the patient's experience and behavior, flexibility and communication are essential throughout the treatment course. The following techniques for treating pain may be used alone or in combination; there are no hard rules which guide choice of technique. Generally, the techniques discussed earlier are used with children whose pain is primarily organic and the techniques discussed later are for children whose pain has a major psychogenic component. But obviously it follows from the earlier discussion of complexities of pain that a child with organic pain might benefit from psychotherapy, while a child with no organic basis for pain might be given medication during the course of treatment.

Medication

The most frequent response to a child in pain, especially if an organic component is obvious, is to prescribe medication. The main problem with this approach is the use of "half-way measures," giving a type or amount of medication that does not afford adequate relief. The child quickly learns that, in effect, he has been deceived. No longer able to trust the medical staff, the child experiences increased anxiety and then may develop a variety of reactions, including hysterical behavior, depression and withdrawal, refusal to cooperate or to eat, and occasionally even psychotic symptoms.

Every pediatrician knows that there are wide individual differences in experiences of and reactions to pain. For instance, a very anxious child will require more medication than a relaxed child, and a child with many previous hospitalizations may need either more or less medication, depending on his previous experiences. Yet many physicians ignore this knowledge and prescribe doses based only on the child's age or weight. It is a good rule of thumb to know that a child expects pain medication to take away most or all of his pain. Failure to achieve this result indicates a need for a change either to a stronger medication, a higher dosage, a different route of administration, addition of another drug, or perhaps psychological intervention to help the child achieve an emotional state in which the drug can have maximal effect.

In cases of chronic or prolonged pain, it is often a mistake to order medication to be given as needed or requested by the child, maintaining certain time intervals. Some children conclude that they must be in severe pain in order to get medication. Then, following known laws of learning, these children consciously or unconsciously exaggerate their pain for fear that otherwise medication will be withheld. In such instances, it is often better to give adequate medication according to a fixed schedule, regardless of pain complaints. Then, in the context of experiencing relatively continuous comfort, patients will usually be more willing to cooperate with the physician in planning gradual withdrawal of medication.

Communication and Coordination with Staff and Family

The physician must take time to explain basic principles of pain medication to all persons closely involved with the patient. Otherwise, unwitting sabotage may occur. A busy nurse may delay 10–20 min in administering medication prior to a painful procedure, thus depriving the child of the full benefit of the medication. As an example, if a child is delayed in going to physical therapy for debridement of burns, the physical therapist's schedule will suffer. However, 1 day of delayed scheduling will, in the long run, prove much less troublesome than many days or weeks of trying to work with a frightened child who does not trust or cooperate and whose anxiety precludes being able to distinguish those aspects of physical therapy which may hurt from those which are painless. With such children, the therapist must probably devote much time to reassurance, cajoling, and explanation, thus having even less time for treatment in each session and further prolonging the total treatment time. In other words, if the physical therapist elects to proceed before medication has taken effect, the schedule for that day will remain intact, but the trauma to the child will take its toll on future sessions. Obviously the same principles are true for nurses and other staff who may treat a child for whom premedication is ordered.

The patient's family may also engage in unwitting sabotage if they are not familiar with such elementary principles as the child's need to trust the staff and the fact that the potency of any medication is related to the patient's faith in its effectiveness. Thus, it is important to provide explanation and reassurance to family members who might otherwise communicate to the child their fears of addiction, their dislike of such side effects as drowsiness, or their own previous idiosyncratic negative experiences with a particular medication.

Occasionally, family members have moral or religious convictions that result in opposition to adequate pain medication. They may feel that suffering is the will of God to be borne gladly, or that suffering is part of reality which the child must learn to accept in order to become a mature adult. They may feel that complaints of pain indicate weakness of character or that children deserve to suffer if they have caused their own pain, e.g., by starting a fire in which burns occurred. Like some professionals, they may fail to appreciate individual differences in response to painful stimuli, or they may even doubt that some children feel pain. Just as with the professional staff, the physician who takes a few minutes to explore and clarify these issues will usually save a great deal of time in the long run.

It is often possible to improve the situation if the physician encourages communication between the family and the nursing and paramedical staff. Then it may be quite easy to determine, for example, whether the child is more anxious when the parents are present than when they are absent. Such information permits rational decisions about whether parents should be present or absent during treatment procedures, when and how long they should visit, and so on. If the child is in a hospital, hopefully visiting rules— even in the intensive care unit—are flexible so as to allow physicians and staff to utilize their knowledge about parent-child relationships. Even if it seems best for the parents not to be with a particular child during painful treatments, their comforting presence at other times and their participation in routine care may reduce the child's baseline anxiety enough to enhance comfort and cooperation during the treatment procedure.

Communication with the Patient

Except for infants, children usually benefit from explanation, unless their anxiety level is very high. If they have some understanding about their disease, the need for treatment, the rationale for a particular treatment, the specific treatment methods to be used, and the sensory and motor experiences to expect during and after treatment, they will probably be more calm and more able to cooperate. Likewise, if they understand the value of pain medication, they may be more willing to take bad-tasting medicine or tolerate injections.

The general goal is to be honest, but not to overwhelm the children with information that is irrelevant to them. Most children do not need to know details of operative procedures which will be performed under general anesthesia. They do, however, need to know what procedures will be done before surgery and why they are necessary. They also need to know what they are likely to feel after surgery, what postoperative procedures will be, where they will be (recovery room, intensive care unit), whether parents will be with them, how their bodies will look, and what limitations (e.g., bed-rest) and demands (e.g., coughing) might be placed upon them. For some children, this kind of cognitive mastery is such an important coping mechanism that they want a running commentary from the doctor or nurse throughout each procedure. They may cooperate much more if they know what each step will be.

Some children also benefit from the feeling of mastery and control that comes with having choices. Since treatment is mandatory, one might think there are no choices. But children who require injection can often be allowed to choose the injection site, and children who need a series of exercises can usually have some input into which exercises are done first. The resulting sense of control allays anxiety and this, in turn, decreases felt pain and enhances cooperations.

Communicating with children who have pain may also help determine which of several simple methods of pain control will be most helpful. Some children respond positively to simple relaxation methods, such as deep breathing or concentrating on relaxing certain body parts. Others, however, find these suggestions aversive. Some children benefit from distraction techniques (e.g., talking about something else, pretending to be in another place), but one must not assume that distraction will help all children. When cognitive mastery is a central coping device and the child needs to know everything that is being done, then attempts at distraction will only heighten anxiety. For some children with chronic pain, distraction techniques may be interpreted as meaning that the staff does not believe they really feel pain, or that the medical staff is deceiving them.

Hypnotherapy

Some children respond dramatically to hypnotherapy for pain relief, but the therapist must take care to use only those methods which are acceptable to particular children at particular times. Thus, hypnotic procedures involving fantasy or progressive relaxation may be very helpful to some patients and useless to others. Some patients may respond best when the hypnotherapist encourages continued alertness and focuses directly on altered sensation, e.g., letting the painful area feel numb or be filled with comfort until there is no room left for pain. Hypnotherapy is a method which requires special training to guide the patient into an altered state of consciousness. It goes beyond the simple distraction and relaxation methods and it should be utilized only by staff who are competent in its use. The same requirement of special training pertains to all the pain control methods discussed in this chapter.

The mechanism by which hypnotherapy reduces pain perception is complex and not fully understood. It appears to be related to dissociation of awareness of the pain, although recent research provides convincing evidence that the pain is experienced out of awareness. Thus, physiological indications of pain are present at the same time the subject is reporting no pain. The most thorough discussion of this subject, including hypnotherapy for relief of pain in children, is contained in the recent book by Hilgard and Hilgard (18). Other hypnotherapists also report that children may achieve pain control through hypnotic techniques (7, 14, 15, 21, 22, 27, 28).

Biofeedback

Biofeedback is another method in which patients may reduce pain through various relaxation and imagery techniques. They are taught to attend to machines which provide continuous information about muscle tension, body temperature, and other physical states which produce or are related to pain. Thus patients become much more aware of the precursors of pain and the milder pain states which can be most easily controlled. When pain is severe, they learn to perceive mild pain decrements which might otherwise go unnoticed and they then experience decrements in anxiety which contribute to further pain relief. More clearly than other methods, biofeedback shows patients they have considerable control over increasing or decreasing their pain. For patients who are relieved by such knowledge, biofeedback may be very useful, especially for certain types of pain such as migraine and tension headache and other stress-related pain. However, if a patient's psychological problems include aversion to taking responsibility for pain, biofeedback probably will not be useful. More research is needed reporting the efficacy and uses of biofeedback with children in pain.

Behavior Modification

This form of psychotherapy involves several approaches to changing pain behavior or experience by systematically changing the environmental response to the patient. The assumption here is that one or more aspects of the environment reinforce the pain and thus maintain and strengthen it. For example, parents of the child who complain of pain may be especially attentive, spending extra time, eliminating usual chores, allowing school absence, and even giving gifts as an expression of sympathy and concern. Other relatives and friends may similarly reward pain behavior, teaching the child that his pain makes him special and deserving of all sorts of pleasant experiences that would not otherwise be his due.

The picture may be complicated by more pathological reinforcers. A child may sense that his parents want to infantalize him and somehow dread his growing up. The child can meet the parents' need by becoming an invalid, thus prolonging the parents' care-taking behavior and avoiding the chance thatr increasing independence might produce parental anger or might even destroy the parents. Other possible dynamics include the child's wish to compete for attention with a sick parent, or even to maintain a relationship with a parent or other significant person who has died.

In all these situations, the children experience conflict regarding maintenance of pain behavior and sometimes overtly express an unwillingness to give it up. Behavior modification generally involves environmental change whereby the child is reinforced for age-appropriate, healthy behavior rather than for pain behavior. Thus special gifts and visits might be arranged when the child diminishes his pain complaints and he might be denied TV or other entertainment when he exhibits severe pain symptoms. In this method, consistency is the key to success, all people must relate to the child the same way all the time.

Failure may result from a doting grandmother who thinks the program is cruel and secretly continues to reinforce pain. The situation may become virtually impossible if a parent consciously or unconsciously refuses to cooperate, perhaps insisting that there really is an organic problem when none exists, or struggles to maintain a symbiotic identification with the child's invalidism. The parents may be the unwitting victims of passive/aggressive behavior in the child, and they may not be able to develop sufficient objectivity because of their own anger. In such cases, where parental counseling fails, the only solution may be to temporarily remove the child from his home and carry out the program in a controlled environment, such as a pediatric or psychiatric ward. The separation not only allows a chance for the child to change, but also provides a period of relief in which the parents may begin to grasp their own pathological involvement and may choose psychotherapy for themselves.

Other Forms of Psychotherapy

Some children may benefit from individual psychotherapy—either verbal or play therapy—in which the goals are to gain insight into pain behavior, increase motivation to change, and try out new behaviors which are more consistent with gradual maturity and independence. Therapy of this kind may last a few weeks or may span several years. Parents and other family members may be treated concurrently, either separately or together in family therapy. Specific techniques will vary widely, depending on the patients' psychological problems and the theoretical position of the psychotherapist.

EVALUATION OF TREATMENT RESULTS

There are no conclusive data comparing the efficacy of these techniques and it is sometimes very difficult to be sure that a child's improvement would not have occurred without any treatment at all. Certainly these questions point to the need for much research.

Some children fail to achieve pain relief, even after several treatment methods have been attempted, and the reason for failure may or may not be understood. Parental sabotage has already been mentioned. We have also mentioned failure to understand and carry out prescribed treatment, even though motivation is present. In addition to medication, behavior modification is often poorly understood and incorrectly applied. Clearly, it is not appropriate to dismiss a treatment as ineffective simply because one is told it has been tried without success. Very specific details must be obtained in order to determine whether the treatment was really given an adequate trial.

In a few cases, the child receives an adequate trial of every conceivably appropriate treatment and still has no pain relief. Usually there is a psychological issue which simply cannot be resolved. For example, a child with an illness which may be perceived as terminal may exhibit pain behavior which seems excessive and which does not respond to treatment. Such a child may equate lack of pain with threatened amputation or even with death, perhaps having heard people rejoice that relatives who died were at last free of pain or that death was God's way of taking away pain. The child reasons that he must have pain if he wants to stay alive and his beliefs may be extremely difficult to change. A few children have a conscious or unconscious need to suffer pain because of real or imagined guilt and they, too, may resist all attempts at relief. Other children come to believe that people in pain are special in the eyes of God and they insist on continuing their sacrifice, perhaps reinforced by religious teachings and deep faith which is the center of their lives.

In such cases, moral and ethical issues cannot be ignored. We might ask whether in specific instances the child may not be better off with some pain than without it. We might also ask whether, for some children, the alternatives to pain may be worse than the pain itself, and whether our insistence on continued efforts at pain relief may have no chance of shifting the balance. In some cases it may be most merciful if we work with the pain rather than against it. We then try to place the child in a milieu—at home or elsewhere—in which people do not react to pain with fear or anger but rather with some measure of understanding and compassion. Such a setting may, in cases of primarily psychogenic pain, allow the patient to be at least a minimally responding, active, and productive human being.

REFERENCES

1. Apley, J. and Hale, B. Children with recurrent abdominal pain: How do they grow up? *Br. Med. J.* 3, 7-9 (1973).
2. Apley, J. A common denominator in the recurrent pain of children. *Proc. R. Soc. Med.* 51, 49-50 (1958).
3. Apley, J., Haslam, D. & Tullock, G. Pupillary reaction in children with recurrent abdominal pain. *Arch. Dis. Child* 46, 337-340 (1971).
4. Apley, J. The child with recurrent abdominal pain. *Pediatr. Clin. North Am.* 14, 1-6 (1967).
5. Apley, J. *The Child with Abdominal Pains.* Blackwells Scientific Publ., Oxford, 1959.
6. Berger, H.G. Somatic pain and school avoidance. *Clin. Pediatr.* 13, 819-826 (1974).
7. Bernstein, N.R. Observations on the use of hypnosis with burned children on a pediatric ward. *Int. J. Clin. Exp. Hypnosis* 13, 1-10 (1965).
8. Carmichael, L. *Manual of Child Psychology,* 2nd ed. John Wiley & Sons, New York, 1954.
9. Christensen, M.F. and Mortensen, O. Long-term prognosis in children with recurrent abdominal pain. *Arch. Dis. Child.* 50, 110-114 (1975).
10. Editorial: Do little bellyachers grow up to become big bellyachers? *Br. Med. J.* 5, 459-460 (1975).
11. Eland, J.M. Children's communication of pain. Master's thesis, University of Iowa, 1974.
12. Eland, J.M. and Anderson, J.E. The experience of pain in children, in *Pain: A Source Book for Nurses and Other Health Professionals.* A.K. Jacox, ed. Little, Brown, & Co., Boston, 453-473 (1977).
13. Friedman, R. Some characteristics of children with "psychogenic" pain. *Clin. Pediatr.* 11, 331-333 (1972).
14. Gardner, G.G. Childhood, death, and human dignity: Hypnotherapy for David. *Int. J. Clin. Exp. Hypnosis* 24, 122-139 (1976).
15. Gardner, G.G. The use of hypnosis in a pediatric setting, in *Psychosocial Aspects of Pediatric Care,* E. Gellert, ed. in press.
16. Gildea, J.H. and Quirk, T.R. Assessing the pain experience in children. *Nurs. Clin. North Am.* 4, 631-637 (1977).
17. Haslam, D.R. Age and the perception of pain. *Psychonomic Sci.* 15, 86-87 (1969).
18. Hilgard, E.R. and Hilgard, J.R. *Hypnosis in the Relief of Pain.* William Kaufman, Los Altos, Calif., 1975.
19. Hooker, D. *Evidence of prenatal function of the central nervous system in man, in On the*

Evolution of the Human Brain. J.A. Leclure, ed. American Museum of Natural History, New York, 1958.

20. Jacox, A.K. *Pain: A Source Book for Nurses and other Health Professionals.* Little, Brown, & Co., Boston, 1977.

21. McCaffery, M. *Nursing Management of the Patient with Pain.* J.B. Lippincott, Philadelphia, 1972.

22. LaBaw, W.L. Adjunctive trance therapy with severely burned ●hildren. *Int. J. Child Psychother.* 2, 80-92 (1973).

23. LaBaw, W.L., Holton, C., Twewll, K. and Eccles, D. The use of self-hypnosis by children with cancer. *Am. J. Clin. Hypnosis* 17, 233-238 (1975).

24. McGraw, M.B. *The Neuromuscular Maturation of the Human Infant.* Reprint ed. Hafner Publ., New York, 1966.

25. McGraw, M.B. Neural maturation as exemplified in the changing reactions of the infant to pinprick. *Child Develop.* 12, 11 (1941).

26. Mennie, A.T. The child in pain, in *Care of the Child Facing Death.* L. Burton, ed. Routledge & Kegan, Paul, London, 1974.

27. Olness, K.N. and Gardner, G.G. The uses of hypnotherapy in pediatrics: A review. *Pediatrics,* in press.

28. Olness, K. In-service hypnosis education in a children's hospital. *Am. J. Clin. Hypnosis* 20, 80-83 (1977).

29. Oster, J. Recurrent abdominal pain, headache and limb pains in children and adolescents. *Pediatrics* 50, 429-436 (1972).

30. Peiper, A. *Cerebral Function in Infancy and Childhood.* 3rd ed. Consultants' Bureau, New York, 1963, pp. 29-33, 539-541.

31. Poznanski, E.O. Children's reactions to pain: A psychiatrist's perspective. *Clin. Pediatr.* 15, 1114-1119 (1976).

32. Schultz, N. How children perceive pain. *Nurs. Outlook* 19, 670-693 (1971).

33. Shirkey, H.C. *Pediatric Therapy.* C.V. Mosby, St. Louis, 1972.

34. Smith, R.M. *Anesthesia for Infants and Children.* C.V. Mosby, St. Louis, 1963.

35. Swafford, L.I. and Allan, D. Pain relief in the pediatric patient. *Med. Clin. North Am.* 52, 31-36 (January 1968).

36. Winter, S.T. Recurrent abdominal pain in children. *Clin. Pediatr.* 15, 771-773 (1976).

CHAPTER 10

Pain and the Aged Patient

T. E. HUNT

The second half of the twentieth century has seen an unprecedented growth of the number of elderly individuals within populations of developed nations. This spectacular biological event will probably continue well beyond the year 2000 (7). No less impressive is the discovery that the majority of people reaching the age of retirement can look forward to many years of health (1). Many of the elderly now participate actively in family and community affairs in ways almost undreamed of only a few years ago. In spite of the frequent accumulation of more than one medical condition throughout a life span, most older individuals manage to adequately cope with independent living at least until the approach of the ninth decade (12). Serious health risks and disability appear to be largely delayed until very old age (25). The special aspects of geriatric care would seem to have their greatest relevance to those individuals who are approaching or have reached the eightieth year.

Progressive aging has been found to be accompanied by profound changes, not only in physiological reserves (21), but also in the clinical features of disease (3). Atypical presentation of illness, a hallmark of geriatric medicine, coupled with diversity of physical and mental status, creates a clinical intrigue unmatched in most other areas of medical practice. One of the more fascinating unusual manifestations in aged patients is that of *pain*. Recognition of unaccustomed symptoms and signs in association with a wide variety

143

of painful states in the aged, will become an increasingly necessary skill of practitioners in a society of increasingly larger proportions of older citizens.

DIAGNOSTIC CONSIDERATIONS

Consideration of pain in the very old patient should be approached under two major premises.

1. Age-related alterations of pain perception and the manifestation of noxious stimuli.
2. Clinical problems in the aged individual.

Age-Related Alterations

Pain perception and recognition and the recognition of noxious stimulation may be profoundly altered in the aged. The older person may complain bitterly of small and niggling or rheumatic types of pain. On the other hand, in diseases usually associated with almost catastrophic pain, the aged individual may experience only minor discomfort or perhaps no pain at all. Not infrequently the onset of an acute lesion in the elderly may be heralded by just a sudden change in behavior or the onset of confusion. Up to 50% of acute myocardial infarctions occur without pain in aged patients (19, 24). This is particularly so after the age of 80 (5). Mild abdominal discomfort and tenesmus have been the sole presenting symptoms prior to irreversible shock and death due to mesenteric artery occlusion with acute gangrene of the bowel. Agitation and noisiness in the normally quiet patient who has advanced organic brain syndrome (dementia), is not infrequently a warning of new lesions, which we would expect to be painful. Any sudden change in behavior in these patients should be recognized as a sign of physical illness, and this may very often be painful.

Reliance in aged patients cannot be placed upon signs of inflammatory disease which frequently would accompany painful states in younger individuals. Immunologic and inflammatory responses are often markedly depressed in the older individual, to the extent that fever may be absent and there may be none of the usual local signs of inflammation. For example, regional lymphadenitis is an infrequent accompaniment to local infection. The masking of responses is not unlike that occurring in hypercorticism, i.e., the rigidity and rebound tenderness may be absent in acute peritonitis associated with bowel obstruction. Sweating in the aged is a hint neither to underlying pain nor to fever associated with painful inflammatory states. Very old patients do not respond as readily by sweating to rises in body temperature, nor do they sweat as profusely as do younger individuals (9).

Referred pain may be much more prominent in the elderly than pain at the site of the lesion. Anderson (2) cites the case of the elderly woman with pain in the neck resulting from an unrecognized gastric ulcer. Personal experiences have also included elderly individuals with pain only at referred sites, while the primary lesions *within the locomotor system* have remained painless. For example, as demonstrated by Kellgren and others (13, 17), painful stimulation of the ligaments between L5 and S1 vertebral bodies will produce pain and tender points along the lateral aspect of the ipsilateral leg, as well as local back pain. In several aged patients, referred leg pain has been the only presenting symptom. Local anesthesia into the primary site of degenerative disease at the lumbosacral joint has abolished these individuals' leg pains.

Misinterpretation of pain by the patient or insufficient attention to historical detail by the physician, may also lead to confusion. Early neurological dysesthesias associated with subacute combined degeneration of the cord, perceived as sole or heel pain, may lead to an erroneous search for foot pathology.

The basic mechanisms of these age-related changes in pain perception have not been elucidated. Nerve conduction times and velocities decrease with the aging process (21). Threshold pain in the arms has been found to be diminished in patients who undergo painless myocardial infarctions (17). Histological studies have revealed a loss of neurons in the thalamus and an increase in neuroglial tissue in the reticular formation with aging (6). Aged human hindbrain substates have been demonstrated to contain increased amounts of 5-hydroxyindoleacetic acid, while serotonin levels remain essentially unchanged (18). This suggests increased activity of serotonin, which is known to be associated with analgesia and enhanced antinociceptive drug potency (15). Further investigation and correlation with present knowledge on this subject is certainly warranted.

Problems Associated with the Elderly Individual

All too frequently the failing memory of the aged patient prevents an accurate historical account of the onset of pain or of the precipitating events. This is especially true of minor traumatic incidents which tend to be rapidly forgotten. Recall of sudden changes in well being or of comfort which is so often relied upon for diagnosis in younger individuals, becomes indistinct. Thus the physician is often erroneously led to believe there has been an insidious onset to a chronic disorder when in fact symptoms are of fairly recent origin and of abrupt onset.

It is also not uncommon for the elderly to fail to report symptoms to their clinical attendants. Unreported "unwellness" is a frequent survey finding among the aged in most communities (3). Symptoms are attributed by patients and relatives merely to the aging process, whereas in fact they may be premonitory indications of impending serious illness. Pain, particularly pain in the locomotor system, is frequently attributed to "old age" and especially to "rheumatism" associated with old age. In reality the origin could include any of a variety of pathogenic causes from trauma to malignant disease.

Unfortunately, it is also not uncommon for the physician to erroneously attribute his patient's symptoms to old age with disastrous delays in achievement of a correct diagnosis and initiation of appropriate therapy. One is reminded of the facetious story of the physician attributing pain in an elderly lady's left knee to old age. To this she responded, "But doctor, my right knee is just as old as the left one!"

Old age is not a disease and there are no diseases attributable solely to the aging process (22). However, there are many medical conditions that are more common in later life or that tend to develop then. Frequently several diseases accumulate over a prolonged life span, adding to the complexity of manifestation of painful clinical syndromes. The presence in an 80 year old of advanced lumbar degenerative joint disease in association with severe diabetic neuropathy, will create marked difficulty in ascertaining the true origin of sciatica-like pain. Physiologically diminished or absent tendon reflexes and reduced peripheral vibration sense, associated with some degree of anemia, may confuse the picture of ischemia of anterior compartment leg muscles due to small vessel disease resulting from diabetes mellitus.

In addition to the memory and cognitive loss associated with chronic organic brain syndrome (dementia), brain function in the aged individual is prone to temporary disturbances resulting from a variety of physical illnesses or their treatment. Acute confusion can be caused by infection, myocardial infarction, congestive heart failure, mild strokes, and other acute illnesses which result in either anoxia or accumulation of toxic products. Injudicious use of drugs, particularly those that are likely to cause hypotension or to have psychotropic effects, commonly produces severe delerium in older individuals. This compounds the problems of diagnosis and management of painful states.

These special influences upon pain of the aging patient can be further clarified by illustrative examples of problems of local and diffuse types of pain. It should be remembered, however, that just as the majority of elderly people are well, so also the majority of pain complaints will be straightforward in their presentations in older individuals. The exceptions to this general observation, however, demand unrelenting clinical vigilance.

PITFALLS IN DIAGNOSIS OF LOCALIZED PAIN

Persisting pains that are localized to specific musculoskeletal areas may be erroneously attributed to rheumatic disorders because the aged patient fails to remember an injurious incident. Hence, traumatic lesions are often unsuspected as causes of chronic joint or bone pain in the elderly. This diagnostic dilemma is frequently compounded by previously recorded incidents of localized arthritis or bony lesions. One key to the accurate solution of such problems is the recognition by either the patient or the relatives of a rather sudden or dramatic increase in localized symptoms or in disability. An older woman with gradually progressive disability from "osteoarthritis" of a hip joint, *suddenly* complaining of more pain or more difficulty in walking should alert her medical attendants to a possible impacted fracture of the femoral neck resulting from a forgotten stumble or actual fall.

A very dramatic similar example occurred in an elderly woman who was known to have had an extreme osteoporosis, but who had managed to walk with only minor discomfort using a single cane. She presented herself for early review because of sudden increase in pain in both hips, severe enough to necessitate use of bilateral crutch supports for ambulation. All hip movements were more limited and painful than on previous examinations, and in recumbency the extended lower extremities assumed positions of external rotation. Radiological studies revealed bilateral femoral neck fractures! She did not recall any type of injury.

Unrecognized trauma may only become evident in some of these cases when eventual investigation of increased walking disability reveals secondary aseptic necrosis of a femoral head.

Both patient and physician may also assume that a known traumatic incident has been of insufficient magnitude to result in serious injury. Very minor stumbles or stresses may result in localized back pain in older women because of the production of "crush" fractures of osteoporotic vertebral bodies. All too often in such circumstances, the onset of symptoms is erroneously attributed to a "traumatic exacerbation" of an assumed underlying degenerative spondylosis. One patient was referred with a "flare-up of spinal arthritis" who was found to have severe spinal osteopenia with two vertebral body fractures. The only stress she had suffered was a simple exertion of hurriedly picking up her overnight suitcase at the local airport!

Another cause of localized pain which may not be easily recognized in an aged individual is that of "failed" treatment. Aseptic necrosis after open reduction and internal fixation is not unusual. In a very old person, gradual resorption of the intervening bony structure of the femoral neck, months or years following pinning of a fracture, may cause protrusion of the pin into the acetabulum with resultant pain. Even acetabular erosions have been found in this type of problem. The aged patient and her physician may erroneously ascribe such discomfort to "posttraumatic arthritis" or they may accept it as a natural consequence of injury and surgery.

One of the commonly "missed" rheumatic problems in the aged group is that of a referred painful shoulder syndrome as a manifestation of cervical spondylosis. Neck complaints may be minimal or have occurred in the forgotten past. Osteoarthritis of the shoulder joint itself is infrequently a cause of limited mobility in older patients. Rotator cuff lesions, however, are common in the elderly, but are almost always accompanied by limitations of particular ranges of shoulder movement and by localized tenderness. Examination of the cervical spine is always indicated in the patient with shoulder complaints, and this is even more essential if these complaints are unaccompanied by any observable immobility of the joint.

Even the localized radicular pain following herpes zoster can create diagnostic difficulties in the older individual. The rash may have disappeared and have been completely forgotten when the patient presents for medical interview because of persisting neuralgia.

Metastatic malignancy as a cause of local pain can never be ruled out in the elderly. Single, presumably negative, radiological studies do not vitiate such a diagnosis. Repeated spinal x-rays remained normal until the last week of life of a patient who died of bronchogenic carcinoma with widespread vertebral metastases. He had presented only with severe back pain 2 months before.

In another patient, both radiologists and clinicians "missed" an erosion of the pedicle of the third lumbar vertebra. The history was that of a lifting back injury which was presumed to have exacerbated obvious degenerative changes superimposed on a previously asymptomatic congenital spondylolysis and spondylolisthesis. Detailed investigations eventually revealed the primary lesion to be a malignant sarcoma in the musculotendonous junction of a gastrocnemius.

PROBLEMS OF DIFFUSE PAIN

Diffuse pain in the older patient may also be difficult to interpret because of an inaccurate medical history, particularly concerning onset and aggravating, as well as relieving, factors. Osteoporosis is probably one of the most common causes in old women of diffuse pain in the back and pelvis, sometimes also the rib cage. This condition is almost universal in women over the age of 80 (18) and is frequently accompanied by the objective finding of bony tenderness.

A sudden onset of widely scattered, severe, centrally located muscular aching in an older individual, especially when associated with marked constitutional signs and symptoms, should arouse suspicion of polymyalgia rheumatica. If such a patient also complains of headaches and is found to have a markedly elevated erythrocyte sedimentation rate, the diagnosis is almost certain. Unfortunately the condition, which is really a giant cell arteritis, is still often misdiagnosed, with sometimes catastrophic results, since occlusion of a branch of the central artery of the retina produces visual impairment and sometimes blindness. The diagnosis is confirmed by arterial biopsy—usually a segment of the temporal artery if headaches are present. Management requires immediate treatment with corticosteroids (4).

Diffuse pains in the lower extremities should direct investigation for possible neuropathy; usually resulting from diabetes or uremia in this age group. Ischemic pains, particularly associated with large vessel disease, are also diffuse over a large segment of an extremity. This is especially true of resting night pain of vascular origin.

Stroke patients may suffer severe diffuse pain throughout the affected side. This is almost always associated with hemianesthesia and responds very often and dramatically to anticonvulsant drugs.

Diffuse limb girdle aching and weakness may result from myopathy. That associated with depressed thyroid function should not be overlooked in an older individual.

Diffuse limb and back pains may be symptoms of depression in the older person. This diagnosis should always be considered if objective evidence of musculoskeletal disorder is absent or if the symptoms appear to overwhelm the physical evidence of disease. In this age group the clinician cannot always rely upon the correlation of radiological evidence of spinal degenerative joint disease and expressed symptoms. Many patients of similar age will present with few if any complaints, although radiographically, findings are just as extensive. Antidepressant therapy is usually followed by marked relief of these patients' symptoms, but it must be pursued for at least 3 or 4 weeks or more.

Painful hypochondriacal states are not uncommon among the younger elderly. However, these seem to diminish in occurrence in very old age. Only a few aged individuals seem to have pain out of proportion to organic disease. Although initially pain may be difficult to explain in some aged patients due to the various factors discussed in the preceding paragraph, inappropriate or affective pain disorders appear to be very less frequent clinical occurrences in very late years.

MANAGEMENT OF PAIN IN THE AGED PATIENT

Since *principles* of pain management in the older patient do not differ significantly from those applying to younger individuals, it is unnecessary to review here every detail of medical, physical, psychological, and surgical treatment used in the control of pain in the elderly. Discussion will be directed therefore towards specific problems arising in the geriatric patient and, particularly, towards pitfalls to be avoided if management of this group of patients is to be successful. A brief comment on the principles of management of the *geriatric patient* should however be appropriate at this point.

Geriatric Care

The management of any clinical problem in the elderly, as in any other group, is based upon initially establishing accurate etiological and functional diagnoses. Only then can appropriate therapy be selected. The very elderly individual is sustained in a delicate homeostatic balance as a result of diminishing physiological functions and, therefore, there is very limited room for therapeutic maneuvering without deleterious adverse results. Because of frequent accumulation of multiple medical conditions over a life span, older individuals will eventually develop multiple complaints and sometimes an extensive list of objective clinical abnormalities. Therapeutic conflicts may then become inevitable as the treatment of one condition may be contrary to that of another. For example, the degree of physical effort involved in successful rehabilitation following a stroke may be impossible as a result of extensive heart disease. Medications required for the management of one condition may interact with those needed for other diseases. The tendency to prescribe potent drug products for symptomatic control only compounds the problem.

These imposed constrictions on therapeutic options in the management of the elderly make it necessary for the clinician to evolve priorities among conditions requiring treatment and to restrict the list of concurrent drug intake. Alternatives to pharmaceutical therapy should be considered wherever possible, e.g., physical therapy, support, splinting, counseling, diet, and simple reassurance.

Successful management of suffering and illness in the elderly is adversely affected by negative attitudes by the attending clinical staff, by overmedication, and by inappropriate use of bed rest. Factors within the patient himself which restrict recovery potential include dementia, extreme age, language and sensory loss, and severe multiple disease (8). The clinician should be realistic in setting therapeutic goals after complete assessment of the whole patient—physically, mentally, and socially. All who are involved in the care of the elderly should also recognize, however, the great potential for recovery, and treatment should be reinforced with positive attitudes of expected improvement whenever appropriate.

The milieu in which treatment is conducted is more important in this than any other age group. The elderly respond best in familiar surroundings among empathetic relatives, friends, and pets. Hospitalization is potentially hazardous for the aged, so its use should be restricted to circumstances in which such facilities are absolutely essential. Even then, hospital admissions should be as short and as restorative in nature as possible.

Often the patient's own home situation may not appear to offer sufficient resources for care at first glance. Consideration should then be given to involvement of visiting nursing or therapy services or organized home care and home help (10).

If available, temporary referral for day care or day hospital utilization can augment care in the home.

Because of the likelihood of multiple complicating problems and because of the potential hazards of drug treatment, older patients require more surveillance and follow-up than do their younger counterparts. It is therefore imperative that the specialist and the generalist cooperate in assuring reviews in office or outpatient clinics at effective intervals. If the patient is unable to attend because of problems of mobility, some type of regular professional visit to the home by either the family physician or visiting nurse should be inaugurated.

It is important, finally, to recognize that there is a time *not* to treat an older individual. Treatment should be withheld when the clinical "abnormalities" reflect merely the aging process; for example, dependent edema in the aged arthritic who sits all day in the wheelchair. Treatment becomes a travesty when it involves the senseless prolongation of life.

Medical Treatment of Pain in the Elderly

Analgesics

All drugs have multiple actions. In younger individuals the desired effects completely overshadow the side or undesirable actions, or the latter only occur at very high doses. In the elderly, adverse reactions occur more frequently, at lower dosages, and may be more prominent. There are really no drugs which are absolutely safe in all aged patients. It is therefore best to start drug treatment, if it is really necessary, with doses smaller than would normally be used for other adults. Gradual increments can then be given until the clinical effect is achieved with minimum dosage.

Simple and single analgesic medications are usually best for the aged patient. Combinations of analgesics or analgesics with hypnotics and sedatives are seldom essential and potentially more hazardous. They should be avoided if at all possible.

Acetylsalicylic acid or acetaminophen are still the safest and the most satisfactory drugs. Both are best given shortly after meals for effectiveness, but if gastrointestinal upsets occur they may be given with food. Enteric-coated forms of ASA may be somewhat less well absorbed in the elderly. Salicylates should be restricted if there are bleeding tendencies and acetaminophen should be withheld in the presence of known hepatic damage.

If antiinflammatory action is required and if such is not being achieved by the intake of salicylates, one of the less toxic nonsteroidal antiinflammatory agents is indicated. In the elderly, it is probably less hazardous to give these agents in place of salicylates or acetaminophen, not in addition to these compounds, as would be prescribed in the younger patient. Ibuprofen has proved to be very satisfactory in relieving joint and other inflammatory pains in the elderly. Confusion and dizziness have each occurred once as side effects in many hundreds of prescriptions for older patients in this writer's experience. Indomethacin is also useful and fairly well tolerated. It appears to act quite satisfactorily in dosages of 50–75 mg *per day* in older individuals. Gastrointestinal symptoms have been somewhat more common with this drug than with Ibuprofen in this observer's experience.

Psychotropic drugs

Very few elderly patients with nonmalignant pain present with a need to be provided with psychotropic drugs *at the same time* as analgesics are prescribed. If anxiety is overpowering it should be separately treated, preferably by measures other than the prescription of very potent tranquilizing drugs. If drugs have to be used it is better to intersperse tranquilizing medication between doses of mild analgesics. Barbituates should not be given to aged patients. Diazepam's popularity is not a reason for its prescription to older patients in whom it can cause confusion and behavioral disturbances. Very small doses of perphenazine or promazine for short periods of time can produce good relief of anxiety in these older individuals, and the latter drug is a good bedtime sedative. Once acute anxiety is controlled, the tranquilizer should be replaced by appropriate counseling, participation in community activities, family affairs, or other nonpharmaceutical measures.

Depression

Pain due to depression is primarily best treated by simple analgesics, counseling, occupational and physical therapy. If these measures alone are unsatisfactory, small doses of mood elevating drugs may be required. There is probably little, if any, place in the care of the aged for the use of monoamine oxidase inhibitors. The tricyclic antidepressants are effective, but are definite cardio-toxins and must be given with great care (11). Doses should be started as small as possible at bedtime only and be gradually increased. It usually takes several weeks for the antidepressant effects to be observable. Constant vigilance against untoward cardiac arrhythmias is essential, and if they develop the drug must be stopped. Lithium is useful for the bipolar form of depression which is much less common in the elderly than the unipolar type.

Psychological and social support

Explanation and reassurance are prime considerations in all forms of medical care. These together with appropriate manipulation of the social situation are equally if not more important than the prescribed analgesic medications in later life. Most types of pain in the aged can be controlled with very simple measures, hence encouragement and positive attitudes towards successful outcome are essential. Most older patients respond positively to being given a simple explantion of the nature of the cause of their symptoms. Once so assured, they frequently reconcile themselves to persisting discomfort with minimal dependence upon medication.

Severe terminal pain

Neoplastic disease is not uncommon in the aged, although sometimes it appears to assume a more benign character. Many very old patients tolerate with amazing composure malignant lesions which would be almost unbearable in younger persons. In a number of these patients, simple analgesics provide surprisingly good control. As the disease progresses and as the suffering increases, a number of oral preparations may prove useful; delaying and perhaps averting the necessity of final resort to parenteral narcotics. An effective "pain cocktail" can be derived by combing acetaminophen and diphenhydramine hydrochloride. Other medications, such as chlorpromazine, can be added to potentiate the effect. These three drugs in combination have been successful substitutes for both morphine and meperidine. More potent oral mixtures providing relief for severe pain include the famous

Brompton Hospital Mixture (London, England) or a combination of morphine. cocaine, and chlorpromazine.

SURGICAL MANAGEMENT OF PAIN IN THE ELDERLY

Surgical measures, apart from local injections of painful tissues, are seldom required in the old patient. Rarely are neural extirpation procedures needed because inappropriate pain is less frequent in these individuals. A point to remember in the few instances when this form of treatment may be considered, is that the usual lack of permanent benefit is not necessarily a serious drawback, since life expectancy in these patients may well be less than the limited expected period of relief.

Injection of local painful tissues, i.e., trigger points, is well worthwhile in the older patient. Satisfactory relief of pain may persist for months, occasionally for years when local anesthetic agents are combined with injectable corticosteroids.

A number of patients with degenerative disease in a hip joint will complain of severe pain and tenderness over the tip of the greater trochanter. Injection, as above, of a tender area often gives marked relief and ability to walk once again. Another useful procedure is the injection of painful interspinous and other intervertebral ligaments. As discussed previously, this often gives dramatic relief of referred pain in the legs.

Prevention of later pain and disability by appropriate initial treatment of trauma is a very important surgical consideration in this age group. The duration of disability and the deleterious effects of delayed rehabilitation resulting from expedient surgery should be weighed carefully against the risks involved in a more prolonged and difficult operation which will enhance earlier mobilization and hasten a return to independence. A specific example of this type of situation is that of the stroke patient who sustains a femoral head or neck fracture on the hemiplegic side. Reduction and fixation by the simple pin and plate types of procedure creates a lesser anesthetic risk than the more complicated and longer operation of replacement arthroplasty with, say, an Austin-Moore prosthesis. However, disability, prolonged immobility, pain and other complications associated with the former method may be far greater than after arthroplasty treatment. The postoperative morbidity and possible mortality in the one must be balanced against the higher immediate surgical risk of the arthroplasty, which by permitting early mobilization reduces postoperative complications as well as the duration of major disability.

Physical Treatment of Pain in the Older Patient

Pain may be relieved by a variety of physical measures, including heat or cold, electrical stimulation, acupuncture, appropriate supporting devices, and early progressive mobilization. Any one of these or combinations of them may be used with or without medical or surgical measures. In the old patient, physical treatment should be considered as a suitable alternative to drug therapy as well as an augmenting form of management.

There are more stringent precautions required in the physical treatment of an older person than are necessary for his younger counterpart. In addition to the problems involved with cardiopulmonary fitness and exercise tolerance, the aged individual must be carefully appraised in terms of sensory perception, hydration, and thermal regulation. Diminished sensation of pain, heat and cold, and deep pressure may result in burning, freezing, or mechanical trauma if a sensory examination has not preceded application of physical modalities. Heating and exercise may produce increased respiration and, hence, water loss in an individual whose hydration is already borderline. Drinking water or fruit juices should always be available in a physical therapy department treating elderly patients. Deep heating can result in hyperthermia because of loss of heat regulating mechanisms. Mild dehydration and mild hyperthermia, resulting from unwary physical treatment, may not be necessarily life threatening, but can produce confusion and negate the value of mobilizing exercises.

Neither heat nor cold should be applied in the region of ischemic tissue. Proximal warming may have some value, as this would hopefully produce vasodilatation of patent collateral vessels, similar to the effect of sympathetic blockade.

Mobilization of involved joints may also relieve pain. For elderly patients, an effective aid to early mobility is the adjustable tilt table (16). It provides safety through varying the degree and placement of support while exercising. Through gradual resumption of the upright position, it provides retention of vasomotor control as well.

Appropriate supportive devices constitute a well recognized measure to relieve pain. The simple procedure of using a walking cane greatly modifies the weight forces upon hips and knees (20). Crutches fitted with horizontal trough-shaped arm supports provide marked relief of weight transfer through hands, wrists, and elbows. Resting splints to protect and support painful joints while asleep add greatly to the comfort of arthritic patients. Proper fitting shoes and foot supports are frequent requirements of elderly patients. Often they may obtain dramatic relief of foot pain on walking and standing, simply through the use of heel wedges or arch supports.

In Summary

In a number of aged individuals, pain may be considerably modified in its perception as a result of physiological age-related changes. Diagnostic difficulties also arise because of various other changes in the older person, e.g., memory loss. The management of the older patient with pain requires consideration of additional age factors, particularly, the hazards of drug therapy. As a result of concurrence of multiple disease processes, priorities have to be established in developing treatment regimes. Great care is necessary less the clinician substitute other forms of disability in the search to relieve suffering.

REFERENCES

1. Anderson, Sir W.F. Geriatric medicine: An academic discipline. *Age Ageing* 5, 193-197 (1976).
2. Anderson, Sir W.F. Geriatrics—Why and how. Presented at the Symposium on Geriatrics, Royal College of Physicians and Surgeons of Canada, Quebec, P.Q., January 1976.
3. Anderson, Sir W.F. *The Practical Management of the Elderly.* Blackwells Scientific Publ., Oxford, 1977.
4. Boyle, J.A. and Buchanan, W.W. *Clinical Rheumatology,* Blackwells Scientific Publ., Oxford, 1971, pp. 434-436.
5. Basu, S., Sinnah, A.T., and McCarthy, S.T. Pain in myocardial infarctions in the elderly. Presented at the Cardiology Seminar, British Geriatric Society, London, October 1977.
6. Brizzee, K.R. Morphometrics, quantitative histology, in *Neurobiology of Aging.* J.M. Ordy and K.R. Brizzee, eds. Plenum Press, New York, 1975, pp. 416-417.
7. Butler, R.N. The doctor and the aged patient. *Hosp. Practice* 13, 99-106 (1978).
8. Coni, N., Davison, W., and Webster, S. *Lecture Notes in Geriatrics.* Blackwells Scientific Publ. Oxford, 1977, pp. 72-82.
9. Foster, K.G., Ellis, F.P., Dore, C., Exton-Smith, A.N., and Weiner, J.S. Sweat responses in the aged. *Age Ageing* 5, 91-101 (1976).
10. Hunt, T.E. and Crichton, R.D. One third of a million days of care at home: 1959-1975. *Can. Med. Assoc. J.* 116, 1351-1355 (1977).
11. Jefferson, J.W. A review of the cardiovascular effects and toxicity of tricyclic antidepressants. *Psychosom. Med.* 37, 160-179 (1975).
12. Lewis, S. *An Assessment of the Need for Community Health Services among the Elderly.* Saskatchewan Dept. of Health, Regina, Canada, 1975.
13. Lewis, T. and Kellgren, J.H. Observations relating to referred pain, visceromotor reflexes and other associated phenomena. *Clin. Sci.* 4, 47-71 (1939).
14. Meema, H.E. and Meema, S. Involutional (Physiologic) bone loss in women and the feasibility of preventing structural failure. *J. Am. Geriatr. Soc.* 22, 443-446 (1974).
15. Messing, R.B. and Lytle, L.D. Serotonin-containing neurons: Their possible role in pain and analgesia. *Pain* 4, 1-21 (1977).
16. Odeen, I. *Functional Training on the Mini Tilt Table.* Ab Grafisk Press, Stockholm, 1972.
17. Procacci, P., Zoppi, M., Padeletti, L., and Maresca, M. Myocardial infarction without pain. A study of the sensory function of the upper limbs. *Pain* 2, 309-313 (1976).

18. Robinson, D.S. et al. Ageing, monamines and monamine oxidase levels. *Lancet* 290-291, 1972.
19. Rodstein, M. The characteristics of non-fatal myocardial infarctions in the aged. *Arch. Intern. Med.* 98, 84-90 (1956).
20. Rosse, C. and Clawson, D.K. *Introduction to the Musculoskeletal System.* Harper and Row, New York, 1970, pp. 85-89.
21. Shock, N.W. Physiological aspects of aging, in *Proc. 3rd Congress of the Association pour l'etude des Maladies de Civilisation.* Ajaccio, Corsica, 1973, pp. 89-111.
22. Smith, W.L. and Kinsbourne, M. *Aging and Dementia,* Spectrum Publ., New York, 1977.
23. Travell, J. and Rizzler, S.H. The myofascial genesis of pain. *Postgrad. Med.* 11, 425-434 (1952).
24. Thould, A.K. Coronary heart disease in the aged. *Br. Med. J.* 2, 1089-1093 (1965).
25. World Health Organization. *Planning and Organization of Geriatric Services.* WHO Tech. Bull. 548, Geneva, 1974.

CHAPTER 11

The Pain Clinic: An Approach to the Problem of Chronic Pain

DAVID B. BOYD
H. MERSKEY
J.S. NIELSEN

WHAT IS A PAIN CLINIC?

The idea of special clinics for the relief of pain has developed since World War II (1, 4). Many centers now have a pain clinic, although its membership can vary from a multidisciplinary assessment center to a single anesthetist. (In the latter case, the term "nerve block clinic" might be more appropriate.) The goal is the same, to relieve pain using the safest and most effective methods available.

The pain clinic is often viewed as a last resort. The typical image in the minds of many patients and physicians is the patient with a terminal illness, probably cancer, who suffers hopeless, excruciating pain. Yet, there are many other aspects.

PAIN

Since pain is the hallmark of underlying disease both to patient and physician, it is obviously important to carry out all reasonable diagnostic maneuvers to obtain the clearest possible insight into what disease process is affecting the patient. Sometimes, the patient's pain is largely, or even wholly, of psychiatric origin (9, 10). It goes without saying that if a specific therapy is available it should be used. However, once the significance of the pain is recognized, it would be ideal for the patient not to suffer it any longer. This would apply to pain of any cause, be it transient, ongoing, or terminal.

WHO RELIEVES PAIN?

Relief of pain is part of the domain of every physician. Each of us approaches it from our own viewpoint and with our own bias. This means that the same patient may get different treatments simply depending on which specialist (or family doctor) he sees. This is not necessarily bad but it does bear looking into. What the patient deserves is the most effective pain relief possible with the least overall cost, in terms of side effects, complications, peace of mind, time, and money.

The best way to choose effective therapy is to have one physician who is primarily responsible and who can weigh the opinions of all the consultants involved. The interchange of ideas that occurs becomes especially important when a long term problem is being considered (15). It is also vital that the patient can relate to one primary physician who can interpret the whole situation. Normally, this would be the family physician, but in practice, unless the family physician is unusually active at the hospital, it is necessary to delegate this role, at the place where investigations and treatment are being carried out, to one of the specialists interested in pain, at least for the phase of active hospital care.

Which individuals should be consulted to sort out a pain problem will vary with the particular patient's problem, but the following disciplines should be considered: anesthesia, neurology, neurosurgery, orthopedic surgery and other surgical subspecialties, psychiatry (8, 14), radiotherapy, physical medicine, internal medicine, dentistry, physiotherapy, psychology, social work, nursing, and pharmacology. From this list, it is most beneficial to choose that array of consultations which suits the problem. For example, a patient with trigeminal neuralgia might best be helped by the opinions of a neurologist, an anesthetist, a neurosurgeon, and a psychiatrist. The bare essentials must include a diagnostician and a therapist. For example, lumbar sympathetic block with anesthetic agents can be useful in diagnosis and prognosis before surgical sympathectomy is considered.

Table 1. Disorders Seen in Pain Clinic

Neurological Disorders
  Nerve lesions
    posttraumatic neuritis
    causalgia
    postoperative neuromas
    amputation stump pain, phantom limb pain
    coccydynia
    scar pain
    nerve entrapments
  Postherpetic neuralgia (shingles)
  Trigeminal neuralgia (tic douloureux)
  Sympathetic dystrophy (e.g., shoulder hand syndrome)
  Painful spastic states
  Thalamic pain

Musculoskeletal Disorders
  Low back pain (spondylitis, arthritis, failed disc surgery, etc.)
  Myofascial pain syndrome (e.g., frozen shoulder)
  Paget's disease (with encroachment on nerves)

Ischemic Disorders
  Peripheral vascular disease (claudication, Raynaud's disease)
  Angina pectoris

Neoplasms
  Direct invasion or compression of painful structures
  Metastases

Psychiatric disorders (3, 5, 21)
  Neurotic illness and mixed depressions
  Headache (some types)

Miscellaneous
  Dental pain
  Myofascial pain dysfunction syndrome
  Tempo-mandibular joint arthritis
  Other facial pain
  Chronic pancreatitis
  Gout

Obscure
  Pain of unknown cause (e.g., obscure abdominal pain)

Table 2. Means of Pain Relief

1. Rest

2. Physical measures
   a. Physiotherapy, exercise
   b. Heat, cold, vibrators, cold sprays, radiation (e.g., short-wave diathermy)

3. Local infiltration with anesthetic agents or steroids

4. Electrical counterstimulation—to skin, nerve, or cord

5. Acupuncture

6. Analgesics
   a. Nonnarcotic
   b. Narcotic

7. Psychotropic agents (11)
   a. Hypnotics
   b. Antidepressants
   c. Tranquilizers—minor and major

8. Detoxification (18) from various combinations of the above

9. Psychotherapy (11)—many forms, including supportive, hypnosis, biofeedback, relaxation, behavior modification

10. Nerve blocks
    a. Temporary
    b. Permanent—pharmacological or surgical

11. Rhizotomy, cordotomy (13)

12. Stereotactic neurosurgery (13)—destruction of thalamic nuclei

13. Hypophysectomy (12)

14. Leucotomy—unilateral or bilateral

15. Radiotherapy

16. Electroconvulsive therapy

17. Other drugs, e.g., steroids, anticonvulsants, chemotherapy, hormones, (or gonadectomy)

WHO ARE THE PATIENTS?

The patients attending pain clinics are a heterogeneous group of all ages with all sorts of problems (5). Ongoing pain is their common feature. A partial list of those disorders which are seen is presented in Table 1, which draws upon our own experiences and those of others (6, 20).

Table 1 illustrates the variety of disorders with which a pain clinic is involved. Note especially, many of the problems are not hopeless, nor do they only occur in old debilitated people.

RELIEF FROM PAIN

Even without altering the basic pathophysiology of pain, physicians are accustomed to relieving it. The things that we do to achieve pain relief vary from simple psychological support and avoidance of aggravating factors to complicated neurosurgery. Table 2 lists the alternatives available.

Some of these are everyday solutions for common problems; others are almost never used. The important thing is to consider the whole range available and to appropriately match the patient and his treatment. The rate of success varies with diagnosis, but, even in the most discouraging population of severely ill patients with terminal malignancies, reasonable relief can often be given. At the very least, the exchange of ideas that occurs through the pain clinic can assure both the patient and the physician that all choices have been considered.

ORGANIZATION OF A PAIN CLINIC

The main model for pain clinics is that of Bonica (1, 4), whose multidisciplinary, highly organized assessment center in Seattle has been widely acclaimed. Essentially, each patient is initially examined by a physician who also assumes responsibility for choosing and coordinating consultations. This same physician acts as a liaison between the patient, the patient's personal referring physician, and the rest of the pain clinic members. He relays decisions back to the patient and referring physician and is in charge of appropriate medical records and follow-up.

Psychological evaluation, conferences, and teaching are functions that vary with the center. There is also a wide variation in the degree of structure affecting the members of pain clinics. The essential aspect is the realization that chronic pain is a multifaceted problem that can best be helped through a multifaceted approach (17).

SUCCESS AND CONCLUSIONS

We doubt that there is any very good measurement currently available to tell how good, or bad, the results may be from pain clinic treatment (19). Epidemiologic studies of chronic pain are in their infancy. The current interest in delineation (9) and measurement (7, 18) of pain is explanation enough to account for the difficulty in knowing what is the natural course of chronic pain with or without treatment (2). A recent follow-up study (16, 17) of chronic pain patients treated as inpatients showed some improvement in

54%. However, 6 months later, only 10% of the initial group were back to work full time. In part, these poor figures reflect the extreme intractability of some chronic pains. By contrast with those who have terminal illness, some chronic pain patients with nonfatal disease are much harder to help. However, from the point of view of the physician dealing with a long and frustrating problem, it would appear that association with other physicians facing the same type of problems could lead to a less disheartened attitude and to an optimal therapeutic approach. The advantage to the patient is clear.

REFERENCES

1. Bonica, J.J. Organization and function of a pain clinic. *Adv. Neurol.* 4, 433-443 (1974).
2. Bonica, J.J. Introduction to symposium on pain. *Arch. Surg.* 112, 749 (1977).
3. Bonica, J.J. Neurophysiologic and pathologic aspects of acute and chronic pain. *Arch. Surg.* 112, 750-761 (1977).
4. Bonica, J.J. and Black, R.G. The management of a pain clinic, in *Relief of Intractable Pain,* vol. 1, Ed. Swerdlow, M., Excerpta Medica, Amsterdam, 1974, p. 116-129.
5. Chapman, C.R. Psychological aspects of pain patient treatment. *Arch. Surg.* 112, 767-722 (1977).
6. McEwen, B.W., deWilde, F.W., Dwyer, B., Woodforde, J.M., Bleasel, K., and Connelley, T.J. The pain clinic: A clinic for the management of intractable pain. *Med. J. Aust.* 1, 676-682 (1965).
7. Melzack, R. The McGill pain questionaire. Major properties and scoring methods. *Pain* 1, 277-299 (1975).
8. Merskey, H. The contribution of the psychiatrist to the treatment of pain. *Adv. Neurol.* 4, 605-609 (1974).
9. Merskey, H. The status of pain, in *Modern Trends in Psychosomatic Medicine,* vol. 3. O.W. Hill, ed. Butterworths, London, 1976, p. 166-186.
10. Merskey, H. Psychiatric management of patients with chronic pain, in *Persistent Pain, Modern Methods of Treatment,* vol. 1. Ed. S. Lipton, Grune and Stratton, New York, 1977, p. 113-128.
11. Merskey, H. Psychological aspects of pain relief, hypnotherapy, psychotropic drugs, in *Relief of Intractable Pain,* Ed. M. Swerdlow, 2nd ed. Excerpta Medica, Amsterdam (1978), p. 21-48.
12. Moricca, G. Chemical hypophysectomy for cancer pain. *Adv. Neurol.* 4, 707-714 (1974).
13. O'Neal, J.T. Managing chronic pain. *Am. Fam. Phys.* 10, 74-80 (1974).
14. Pilowsky, I. The psychiatrist and the pain clinic. *Am. J. Psych.* 133, 752-756 (1976).
15. Simpson, D.A., Saunders, J.M., Rischbieth, R.H.C., Rees, V.E., Burnell, A.W., and Cramond, W.A. Experiences in a pain clinic. *Med. J. Aust.* 1, 671-675 (1965).
16. Swanson, D.W., Floreen, A.C., and Swenson, W.M. Program for managing chronic pain. II. Short-term results. *Mayo Clin. Proc.* 51, 409-411 (1976).

17. Swanson, D.W., Swenson, W.M., Maruta, T., McPhee, M.C., Program for managing chronic pain. I. Program description and characteristics of patients. *Mayo Clin. Proc.* 51, 401-408 (1976).
18. Sternbach, R.A. Psychological factors in pain, in *Advances in Pain Research and Therapy*, vol. 1. J.J. Bonica and D. Albe-Fessard, eds. 1976, p. 293-299.
19. Swerdlow, M. 4 year's pain clinic experience. *Anaesthesia* 22, 568-574 (1967).
20. Swerdlow, M. The pain clinic. *Br. J. Clin. Pract.* 26, 403-407 (1972).
21. Wise, T.N. Pain, the most common psychosomatic problem. *Med. Clin. North Am.* 61, 771-780 (1977).

Index